SHADOW AND LIGHT

JOURNAL

THOUGHTFUL PROMPTS FOR PERSONAL GROWTH

SELENA MOON

ROCKPOOL

CONTENTS

INTRODUCTION

Welcome to the *Shadow and Light Journal* and congratulations on choosing you!

This journal will help you to work on yourself and get to know yourself on a deeper level. All the themes to journal on are things we experience through life and there's a high chance you can relate to a lot of them already, if not all. Actively engaging and putting your thoughts down on paper rather than just thinking about these issues can significantly help you work through them and move forward.

It's easy to sometimes get stuck in thought patterns and although we are always growing by just experiencing life, reflecting on these different themes can help you propel your self-growth and aid you in living a happier and more thoughtful life, as well as help you overcome struggles and view things from a multitude of perspectives you might not have considered before.

The themes are derived from the *Shadow and Light Oracle* deck, which I created for the same purpose: to help people grow and challenge their own thoughts. You can use this journal as a tool to accompany the deck or use it independently; they are both designed to work together as well as individually, it's up to you how you prefer to use them.

Each theme consists of two words accompanying each other, representing a relationship, whether they are dependent on each other or opposing each other; therefore, you will be reflecting on 72 themes overall.

HOW TO USE THIS JOURNAL

This journal contains 72 different themes for you to journal on. Each theme has different prompts to help you reflect and move forward towards self-growth.

Each theme has an affirmation that you might find helpful. You can use these themes to meditate on or write them down on notes to give yourself reminders. You can randomly choose one to repeat to yourself for extra empowerment every day or however you find affirmations useful; it's up to you!

There's a reflection section before the themes where you can start to write down your initial thoughts and things you think you need to work on. It's a great way to get you in the mindset of growth. If you prefer to jump right into the themes instead, you can do so as well.

You can jump in and out of the different themes as you please; there's no need to follow a particular order although you can start from the beginning and work your way through. It's completely up to you how you want to use this journal.

If you have the *Shadow and Light Oracle* cards, you can pull from these to help guide you through the journal. You can pull a random card, read the guidance and then go to the corresponding chapter in this journal and write down your thoughts. You could also flick through the pages or cards of the deck to see which one catches your attention and start journalling on that particular theme. If you are drawn to a specific image, it might be an indication that this is something you need to work on right now.

Some of the themes have an incentive for you to take action; it might be a tip or a prompt to help you in a practical way to move forward on that specific topic.

At the back of this journal you will find a section to write down and reflect on what you have achieved and in what areas you have grown. It's easy to forget sometimes how far you've come and this section will help you to acknowledge your growth.

I wish you love, happiness and growth on your personal journey and I hope this journal will help you with that. Remember, we are all constantly growing and you are already doing so well! The fact that you have picked up this journal shows that you take your journey to self-growth seriously and you are already well on your way!

INITIAL
REFLECTIONS

What do I hope to achieve through this journal?

_____

_____

_____

_____

_____

_____

_____

_____

_____

_____

_____

_____

_____

_____

_____

_____

What are my goals in terms of self-improvement?

_____

_____

_____

_____

_____

_____

_____

_____

My current struggles are:

_____

_____

_____

_____

_____

_____

_____

_____

Other notes:

_____

_____

_____

_____

_____

_____

_____

_____

_____

_____

_____

_____

_____

_____

_____

_____

_____

THEMES

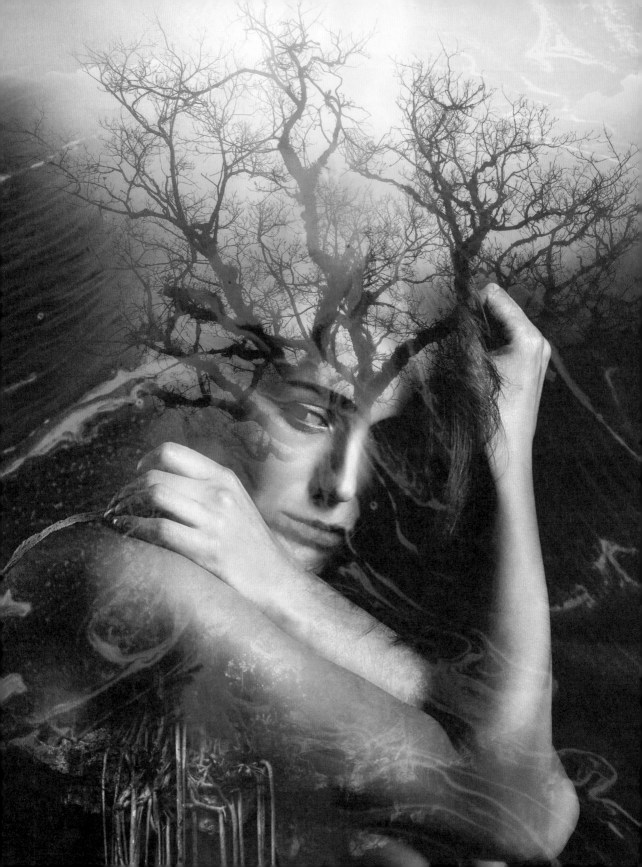

1. Growth | Pain

AFFIRMATION:

*'I embrace the pain and
make way for growth.'*

There can be no growth without pain. We often resist change and growth because it might be painful to let go of what is known to us. We fear what we could become without it. It is easy to fall into the habit of focusing too much on what we leave behind rather than what we have to gain.

✦ Initial thoughts:

_____

_____

_____

_____

_____

_____

_____

_____

✦ What am I resisting in order to achieve the change I'm looking for?

_____

_____

_____

_____

_____

_____

_____

_____

Is there anything I can give up in order to grow? What is it and how would giving this up help?

_____

_____

_____

_____

_____

_____

_____

_____

✦ What in my life would I like to improve, and why?

_____

_____

_____

_____

_____

_____

_____

_____

✦ In what area is there room for me to grow? What can I do to achieve this growth?

_____

_____

_____

_____

_____

_____

_____

_____

✦ What do I need in order to grow?

_____

_____

_____

_____

_____

_____

_____

_____

This is what I have to gain by making these changes:

_____

_____

_____

_____

_____

_____

_____

_____

Tip: Read the list out loud to yourself a couple of times each day, either in the morning or before you go to bed, or take time and meditate upon your list.

ACTION: My next step is:

_____

_____

_____

_____

_____

_____

_____

_____

_____

_____

_____

_____

_____

_____

_____

_____

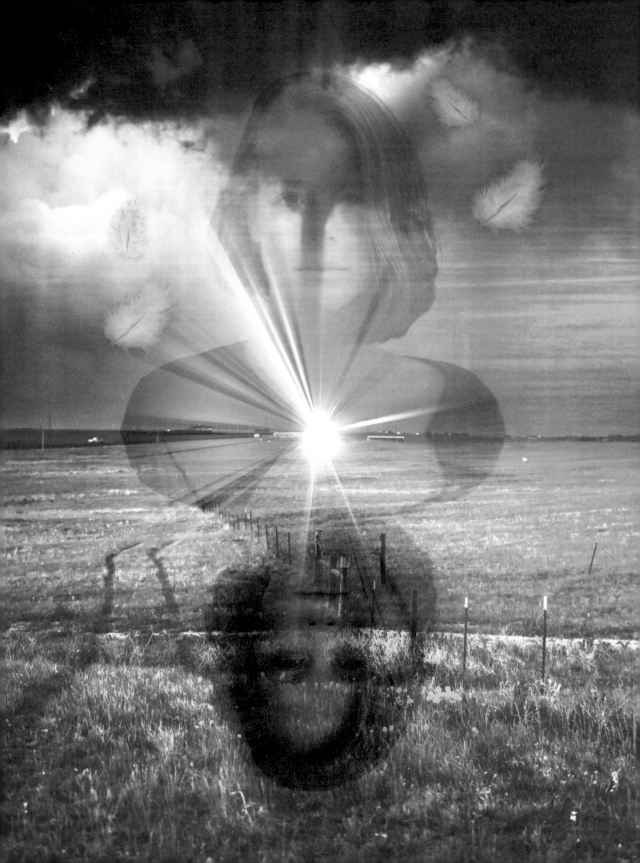

2. Discomfort | Resentment

AFFIRMATION:

'I choose discomfort over resentment.'

We often avoid conflicts or even mentioning our feelings because we fear the discomfort it might cause especially in relationships and even more so in new relationships. It's common to avoid conflicts by focusing solely on the positive things and ignoring negative emotions that need to be addressed just to keep the peace between everyone involved. Direct communication isn't always something that comes easy though, it needs to be learned, and this is an indication for you to practise it. Not communicating directly may instead cause the very thing we fear from communication.

✦ Initial thoughts:

_____

_____

_____

_____

_____

_____

What issues am I currently avoiding to address? Why am I avoiding them?

_____

_____

_____

_____

_____

_____

_____

What, if any, problems am I ignoring in my relationship?

_____

_____

_____

_____

_____

_____

_____

✦ What do I fear by addressing them?

_____

_____

_____

_____

_____

_____

_____

✦ What could I gain by addressing them?

_____

_____

_____

_____

_____

_____

_____

Am I currently experiencing resentment towards anyone? Why?

_____

_____

_____

_____

_____

_____

_____

_____

How will I feel if I don't address these issues?

_____

_____

_____

_____

_____

_____

_____

_____

ACTION: Whenever you notice yourself feeling resentful, write down how you feel and what made you feel that way.

_____

_____

_____

_____

_____

_____

_____

_____

_____

_____

_____

_____

_____

_____

_____

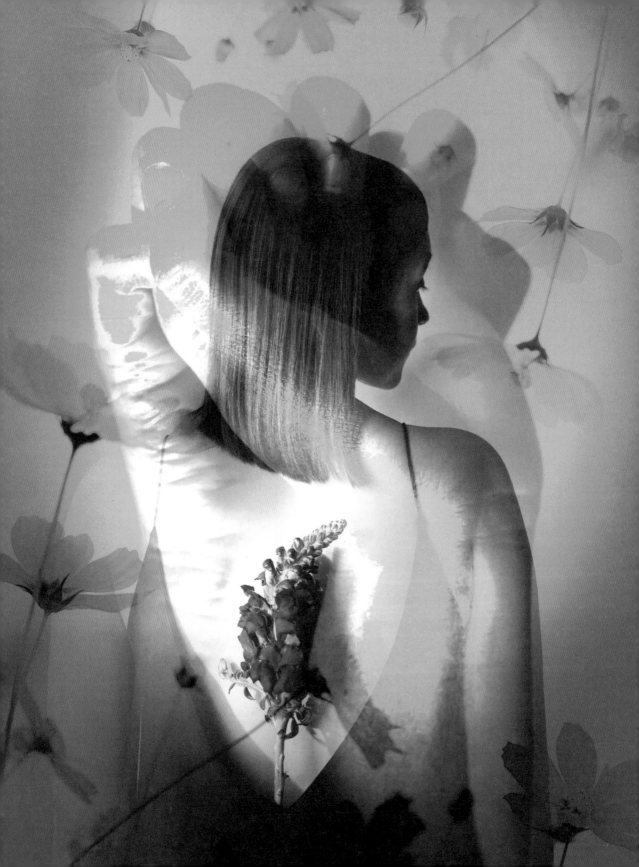

3. Generosity | Egoism

✦

AFFIRMATION:

'I give with a true heart.'

Are you truly giving without expecting anything in return? Are the people in your life doing the same? A lot of transactions we make, whether it be with acquaintances or loved ones, often have a hidden agenda rather than just giving for the sake of giving.

✦ Initial thoughts:

_____

_____

_____

_____

_____

_____

_____

_____

✦ Think about your relationships. Is there anyone who seems to give just to gain something? How does that show?

_____

_____

_____

_____

_____

_____

_____

✦ Think about the times when you have given something to someone, whether it was material things or services. Did you have any hidden agenda other than giving just because you like them? Describe it.

_____

_____

_____

_____

_____

_____

_____

◆ Did you expect anything in return? What were your thoughts when doing this?

_____

_____

_____

_____

_____

_____

_____

_____

_____

_____

_____

_____

_____

_____

_____

◆ What can you do to show your appreciation to your loved ones?

_____

_____

_____

_____

_____

_____

_____

_____

_____

_____

_____

_____

_____

_____

_____

_____

✦ Who would you like to show more appreciation towards, and why?

_____

_____

_____

_____

_____

_____

_____

_____

_____

🌙 **ACTION:** Send a surprise gift or just a simple message to let someone know that they are special to you. Who is the gift or message for, and what will you send?

_____

_____

_____

_____

_____

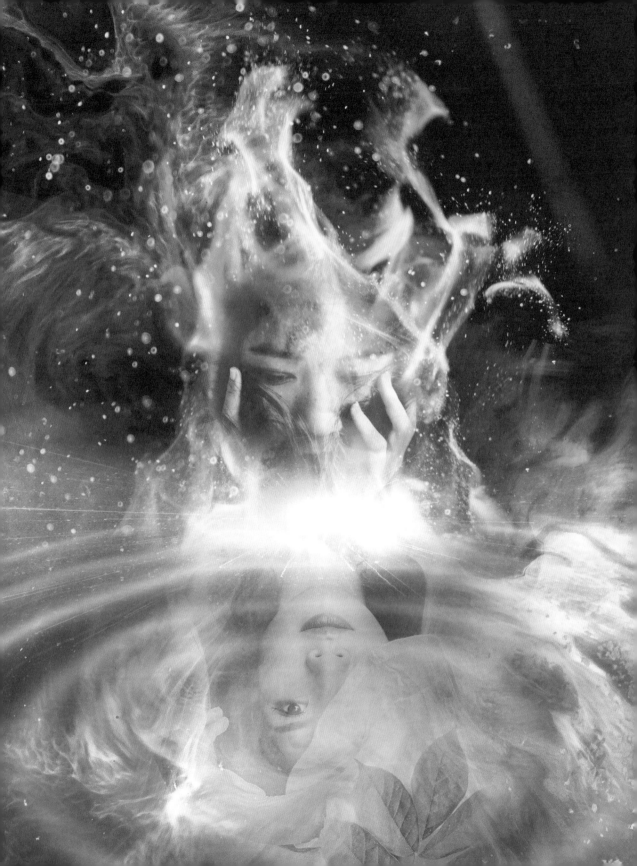

4. Reflection | Overthinking

'I have power over my thoughts.'

Overthinking is extremely common and something most of us do. Things such as asking yourself 'what if?' repeatedly; picturing worst-case scenarios or exaggerating the severity of an issue; constantly looking in the mirror and analysing things about yourself that aren't necessarily true. And the more you do it, the truer they feel to you. So, it's worth taking a step back and starting to think about the things you are telling yourself, what you see might not be what others see.

✦ Initial thoughts:

_____

_____

_____

_____

_____

_____

_____

_____

What is a current struggle you keep replaying in your mind?

_____

_____

_____

_____

_____

_____

_____

_____

_____

_____

_____

_____

_____

_____

_____

What are your 'what ifs'?

_____

_____

_____

_____

_____

_____

_____

_____

_____

_____

_____

_____

_____

_____

_____

Are the things you are replaying in your mind true? What evidence do you have that your thoughts are true?

_____

_____

_____

_____

_____

_____

_____

_____

_____

_____

_____

_____

_____

_____

◇ What might be an alternative truth?

_____

_____

_____

_____

_____

_____

_____

_____

_____

 ACTION: Get a nice piece of paper, perhaps in your favourite colour, and write down these three questions:

1. Do I have proof that what I am thinking is true?

2. What might be an alternative truth?

3. What soothing thing can I tell myself?

Put the paper in a frame and hang it somewhere you can see it, perhaps near your bed where a lot of overthinking might be happening so that every time you start worrying, you can look at these questions and start answering them to calm your mind.

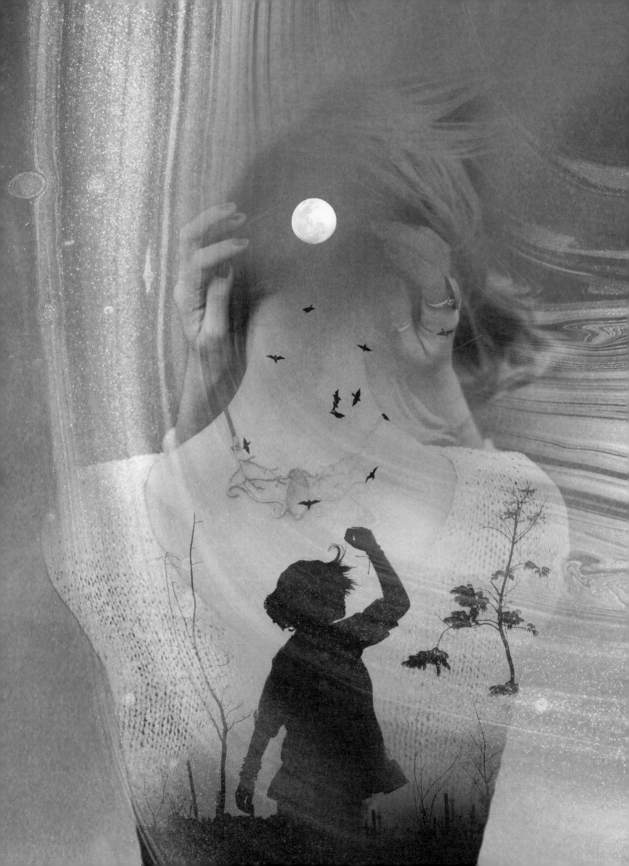

5. Self-doubt | Hope

AFFIRMATION:

'I will give myself a chance to succeed.'

As newborns, self-doubt is not a concept that is yet developed. Even in young children, the thought that they won't be able to do something doesn't occur as much. For example, when a child starts walking they will keep falling over but keep trying until they succeed. This confidence, the notion of never giving up, slowly gets lost over time in a society that constantly compares achievements and everyone's successes are on display. Here is a chance for you to find courage to believe in yourself again.

✦ Initial thoughts:

_____

_____

_____

_____

_____

_____

_____

_____

✦ What is a goal you are currently trying to achieve?

_____

_____

_____

_____

_____

_____

_____

✦ What are the doubts in your mind about this goal?

_____

_____

_____

_____

_____

_____

_____

_____

◆ Why do you want to achieve this?

_____

_____

_____

_____

_____

_____

_____

_____

_____

_____

_____

_____

_____

_____

_____

_____

✦ What keeps you motivated to try?

_____

_____

_____

_____

_____

_____

_____

_____

_____

_____

_____

_____

_____

_____

_____

_____

◆ What are some small steps you can take towards achieving this goal?

_____

_____

_____

_____

_____

_____

_____

_____

_____

_____

_____

_____

_____

🌙 **ACTION:** Choose one item from your list of small steps and take action on it.

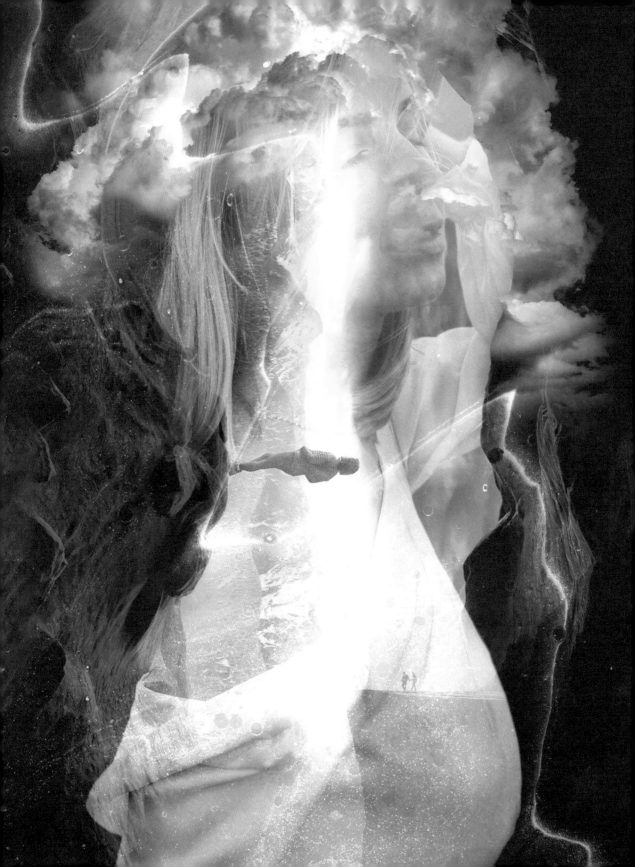

6. Shadow | Light

AFFIRMATION:

*'I see you, pain; I feel you, pain; I give
you permission to move through.'*

Life is a constant roller coaster; nothing is permanent and circumstances change all the time. There cannot be any concept of light if darkness does not exist and there couldn't be any shadows without the light. If the light was constant, we wouldn't appreciate it and we appreciate the dark only because we've experienced the light. If you truly want to enjoy your brightest moments, be brave enough to explore what's in the shadows, so you can blow away any upcoming dark clouds and enjoy the light again.

✦ Initial thoughts:

_____

_____

_____

_____

_____

_____

_____

What do you love in your life right now?

_____

_____

_____

_____

_____

_____

_____

_____

_____

_____

_____

_____

_____

_____

_____

_____

How can you acknowledge and celebrate these things?

_____

_____

_____

_____

_____

_____

_____

_____

What is something that currently clouds your mind?

_____

_____

_____

_____

_____

_____

_____

_____

What steps can you take to acknowledge and work through this struggle?

_____

_____

_____

_____

_____

_____

_____

_____

_____

_____

_____

_____

_____

_____

_____

_____

ACTION: The first step to moving through difficult emotions is to acknowledge them. Practise taking this first step whenever you realise there is some darkness that needs to be dealt with. Use any of the mantras 'I notice that I feel . . .' (or come up with your own that works for you). Fill in the dots with whatever feeling you have noticed. If you don't know exactly what you feel, you can voice that too and just acknowledge that you feel *something* that is uncomfortable.

You can voice this in your head or write it down here if it feels more helpful.

_____

_____

_____

_____

_____

_____

_____

_____

_____

_____

_____

_____

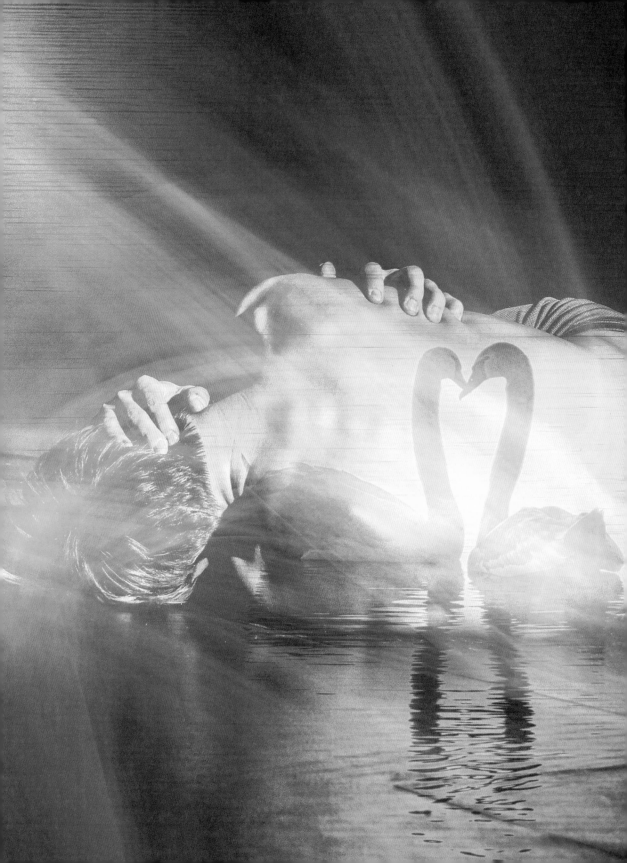

7. Love | Hurt

AFFIRMATION:

*'I accept the hurt that comes with love
as a lesson to help me move forward.'*

There is seldom love without hurt and we must be willing to risk feeling hurt in order to gain the ultimate and exquisite feeling of love – both for others and by others. It's easy to think that love is the reward we get for putting up with the hurt. Use these questions as an incentive for you to turn around that perspective.

✦ Initial thoughts:

_____

_____

_____

_____

_____

_____

_____

_____

◆ What is some hurt you are currently feeling from past love?

_____

_____

_____

_____

_____

_____

_____

◆ What has this hurt taught you?

_____

_____

_____

_____

_____

_____

_____

How can you use this knowledge to move forward in love?

_____

_____

_____

_____

_____

_____

_____

_____

ACTION: Make a list of things that happened that made you feel hurt. Next to each point, write down what this has taught you. Use this list to help you navigate towards better relationships and hopefully less hurt.

_____

_____

_____

_____

_____

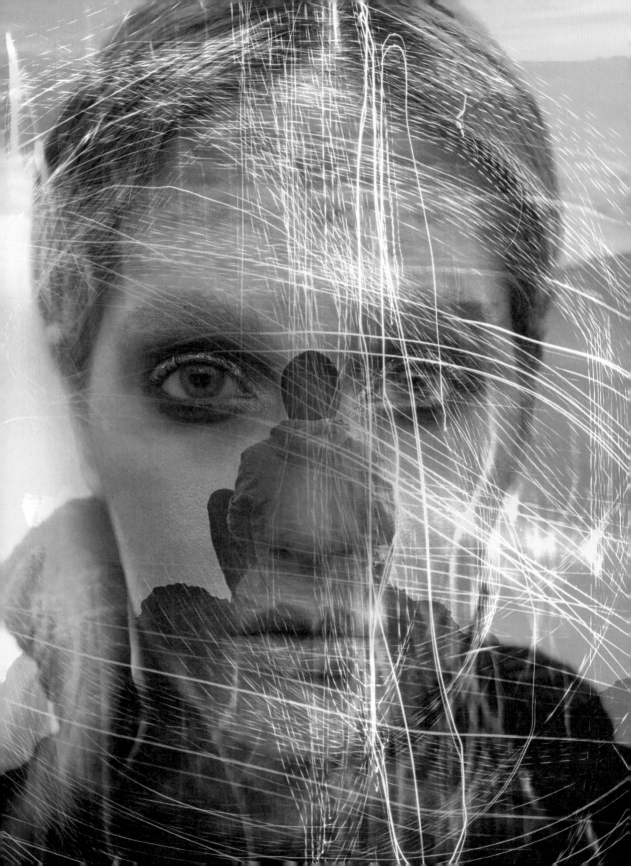

8. Relationship | Solitude

*'I welcome my alone time as
much as my relationships.'*

Relationships and solitude work in symbiosis; strive to keep a healthy balance at a level that works for you. It might not be the same for everyone, some people require more alone time and some don't need as much.

✦ Initial thoughts:

_____

_____

_____

_____

_____

_____

_____

_____

◆ Do you require more alone time or more togetherness, and why?

_____

_____

_____

_____

_____

_____

◆ What can you do to improve the balance between the two?

_____

_____

_____

_____

_____

_____

_____

_____

How can you embrace and enjoy your alone time more?

_____

_____

_____

_____

_____

_____

_____

_____

_____

_____

_____

_____

_____

_____

✦ What fills your heart the most outside of relationships with others?

_____

_____

_____

_____

_____

_____

_____

_____

_____

_____

_____

_____

_____

_____

_____

_____

What can you do to be more present and engaged in your relationship?

_____

_____

_____

_____

_____

_____

_____

_____

_____

_____

ACTION: Fill two separate bowls with activity ideas, one with things you enjoy doing alone (solitude bowl) and one with things you like to do with your partner (relationship bowl). When you feel you need to balance out your time alone and together, pull a note from the bowl you need more of.

If you are single, when you are feeling bored you can revisit your solitude bowl and get tips from yourself on how to feel more joyful. And if you happen to enter a relationship (or are already in one), you can use the solitude bowl to remind yourself to keep doing the things you like to do alone, while also enjoying the things from the relationship bowl.

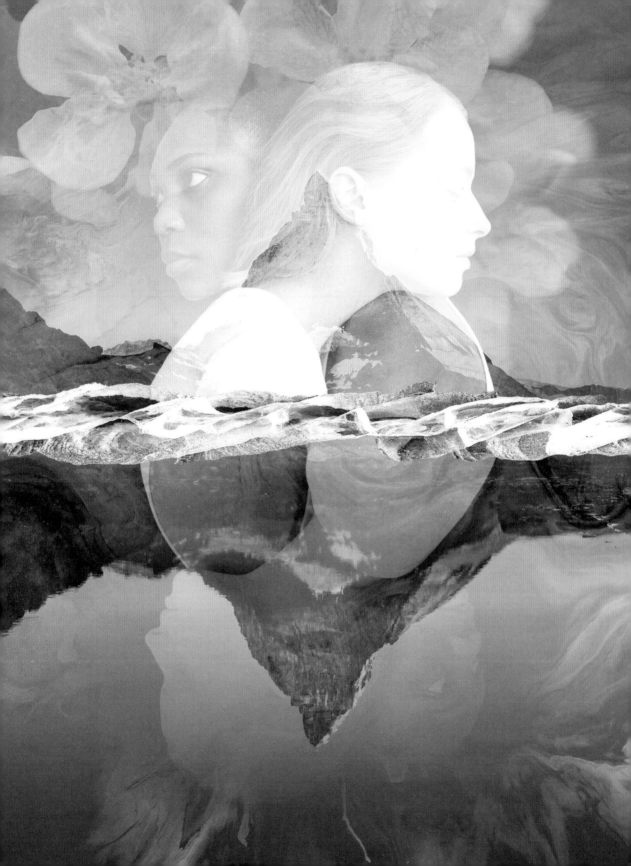

9. Vulnerability | Empathy

AFFIRMATION:

'My vulnerability is my strength.'

Empathy is the ability to truly feel and be with someone in their feelings. To walk together with them on a dark road. It is not standing beside and waving at them but truly being there for them. To hold their hand and drown with them for a moment and be able to feel their emotions with them.

✦ Initial thoughts:

_____

_____

_____

_____

_____

_____

_____

_____

_____

_____

◆ What is something you are currently feeling vulnerable about?

_____

_____

_____

_____

_____

_____

_____

_____

_____

_____

_____

_____

_____

_____

◆ Who would be the person you feel most comfortable sharing this with, and why?

_____

_____

_____

_____

_____

_____

_____

_____

_____

_____

_____

_____

_____

_____

_____

_____

✦ What could you gain from sharing it with that person?

_____

_____

_____

_____

_____

_____

_____

_____

_____

_____

_____

_____

_____

_____

✦ Think about the last time someone shared something sensitive with you. How did it make you feel?

_____

_____

_____

_____

_____

_____

_____

_____

_____

_____

☾ **ACTION:** Next time a close friend asks you how you are, try and stop for a second and not automatically just reply that you're fine if you are not. See if you can be a little more authentic in your response. Start small by admitting it's not the best right now but you are working on it. Or if you are, in fact, extremely happy, try and tell them why – instead of saying 'great', explain the feelings you have, perhaps it's gratitude or love?

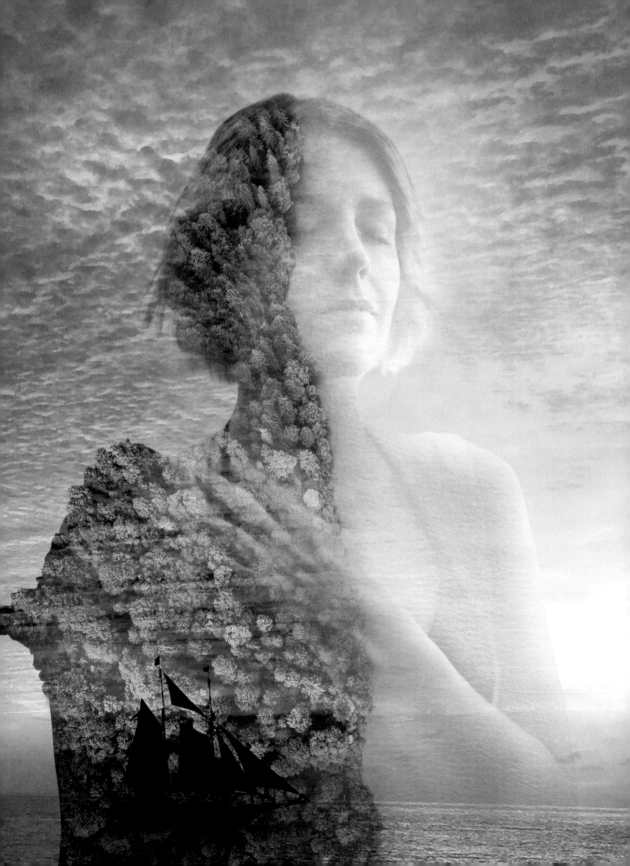

10. Passion | Purpose

AFFIRMATION:

'I trust my passion to lead me to my purpose.'

Passion and purpose are deeply connected. Your purpose is what drives you forward, your motivation, your fuel to your engine. But if you are being asked, 'What is your purpose in life?' you might find that a bit difficult to answer straight away. It is something we rarely reflect over; we just do it.

✦ Initial thoughts:

_____

_____

_____

_____

_____

_____

_____

_____

✦ What are you passionate about?

_____

_____

_____

_____

_____

_____

_____

✦ In what scenario do you feel like time flies and you forget about all the problems and stress in your life?

_____

_____

_____

_____

_____

_____

◆ What motivates you to keep doing those things?

_____

_____

_____

_____

_____

_____

_____

_____

_____

_____

_____

_____

_____

_____

_____

_____

_____

✦ List all the good feelings you have when you do what you are passionate about:

_____

_____

_____

_____

_____

_____

_____

_____

_____

_____

_____

_____

_____

How can you share your passion with others?

_____

_____

_____

_____

_____

_____

_____

_____

_____

_____

_____

_____

_____

_____

_____

_____

_____

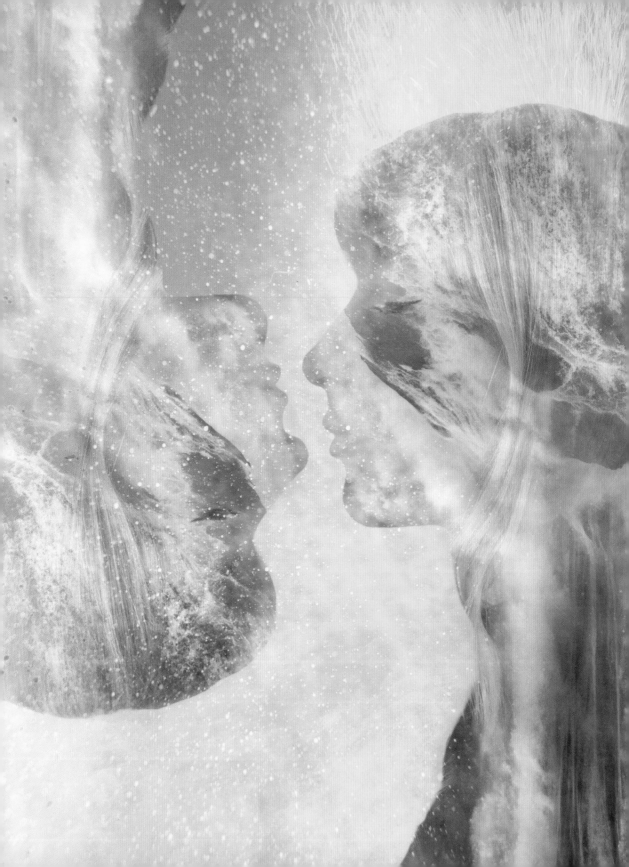

11. Advise | Listen

AFFIRMATION:

*'Deep within, I know how to
solve my own problems.'*

When someone is experiencing hardships, we often like to offer our support in the form of coming up with solutions for them; however, this rarely makes them feel any better and likewise if you're having some issues and people try to suggest solutions you might just feel more agitated. You want to feel heard and you need your feelings to be validated. It is the same for other people too – they might not want to hear your advice right now; they might just want you to listen.

✦ Initial thoughts:

_____

_____

_____

_____

_____

_____

_____

◆ What are some things you can say when someone is opening up to you but not asking for advice?

_____

_____

_____

_____

_____

_____

_____

_____

_____

_____

_____

_____

_____

✦ When do you feel most heard?

_____

_____

_____

_____

_____

_____

_____

_____

_____

_____

_____

_____

_____

_____

_____

How can you offer the same things to others?

_____

_____

_____

_____

_____

_____

_____

_____

_____

_____

_____

_____

_____

_____

_____

_____

✦ How can you express to your friends that you just want them to listen?

_____

_____

_____

_____

_____

_____

_____

_____

_____

_____

_____

🌙 **ACTION:** Next time you seek support from a friend, practise telling them before you start what you would like to hear from them. And next time someone comes to you for comfort, ask them first if they want advice or for you just to listen.

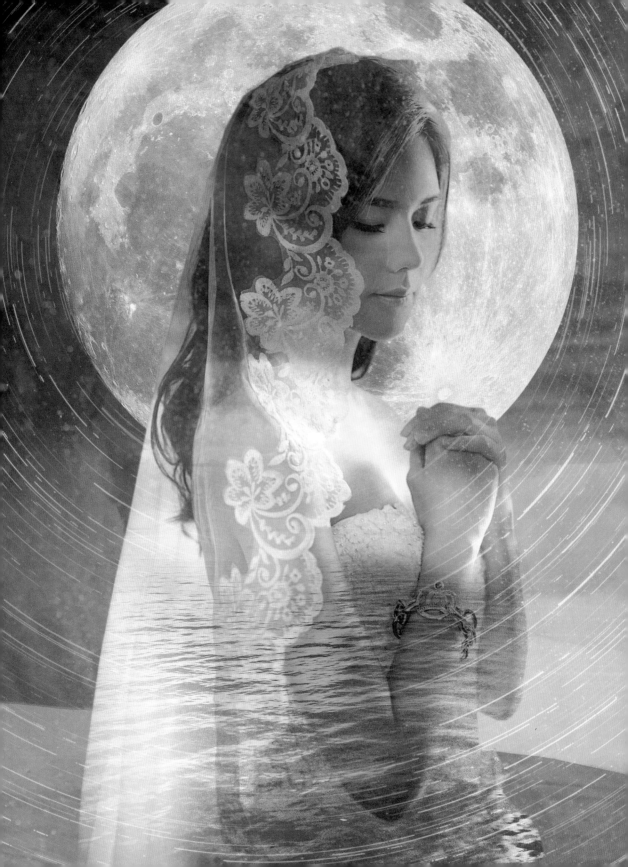

12. Planning | Destiny

AFFIRMATION:

'I am where I am supposed to be right now.'

If planning and destiny were sitting on each side of your scale, which one would weigh more? Are you comfortable with that? Some people believe that everything is destiny and nothing ever turns out a way that it shouldn't, and if we think it does, it was for a reason or a purpose. Sometimes, no matter how much we plan or wish for something, it doesn't come true. Or it comes true in a different way than we expected.

✦ Initial thoughts:

_____

_____

_____

_____

_____

_____

_____

_____

_____

_____

What is something you wished for that didn't come true?

_____

_____

_____

_____

_____

_____

_____

_____

What might your life have looked like now had it turned out the way you'd wished?

_____

_____

_____

_____

_____

_____

_____

What other things would you have missed out on had that happened instead?

_____

_____

_____

_____

_____

_____

_____

What did you gain from your wish not coming true?

_____

_____

_____

_____

_____

_____

_____

_____

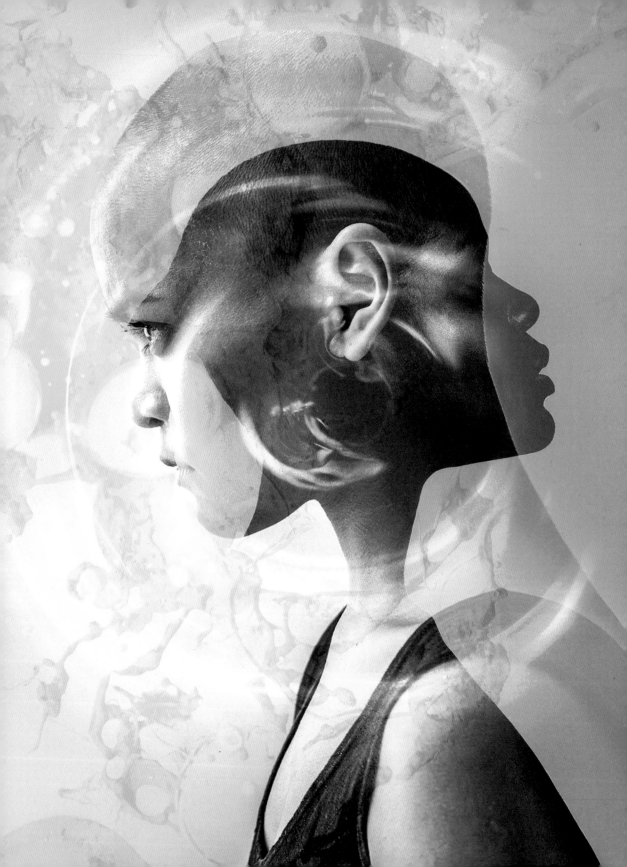

13. Rejection | Maturing

✦

AFFIRMATION:

'I am confident enough to handle rejection.
I do not fear rejection,
it will lead me in a better direction.'

Rejection is something we all experience at certain times in our life and it's a difficult feeling to deal with. It can cause tremendous amounts of pain if we don't learn how to embrace it. When getting rejected it makes us feel inadequate, unwanted and perhaps like we are a failure. It can cause us to fear trying, feeling scared of moving forward and pursuing what we really want.

✦ Initial thoughts:

_____

_____

_____

_____

_____

_____

_____

✦ When was the last time you felt rejected? What happened?

_____

_____

_____

_____

_____

_____

_____

_____

_____

_____

_____

_____

_____

_____

_____

_____

_____

✦ What was your initial response?

_____

_____

_____

_____

_____

_____

_____

✦ What happened after?

_____

_____

_____

_____

_____

_____

_____

✦ What are some soothing things you can tell yourself about the rejection?

_____

_____

_____

_____

_____

_____

_____

✦ How would your life have been different had it not happened?

_____

_____

_____

_____

_____

_____

_____

✦ What did you get to experience instead?

_____

_____

_____

_____

_____

_____

_____

_____

✦ What things are you better off without from the person who rejected you?

_____

_____

_____

_____

_____

_____

_____

_____

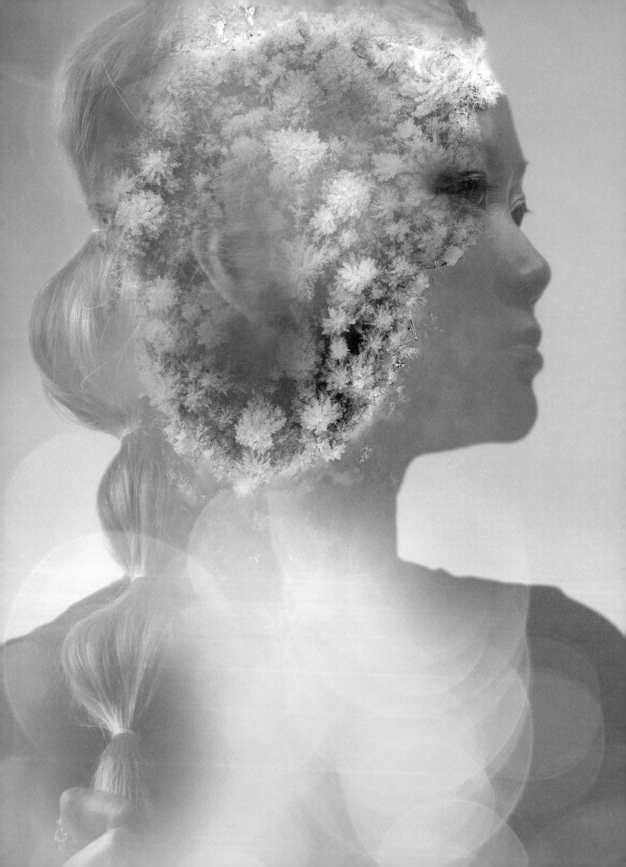

14. Boundaries | Respect

AFFIRMATION:

'I show my respect to others and equally deserve respect in return. I don't need to get better at stating my boundaries, I need to have people in my life who already respect them.'

Setting boundaries with people we love, and even people we don't particularly like, is not always easy. Sometimes you might not even know what your boundaries are straight away if being asked. Here's a chance to start analysing what your boundaries might be and where you would like to implement them more.

✦ Initial thoughts:

_____

_____

_____

_____

_____

_____

_____

What are some boundaries you feel you need to set in your life?

_____

_____

_____

_____

_____

_____

_____

_____

_____

_____

_____

_____

_____

_____

_____

◆ How can you express them to others?

_____

_____

_____

_____

_____

_____

_____

_____

_____

_____

_____

_____

_____

_____

_____

◆ Is there anyone currently not respecting your boundaries? How is this happening and what actions can you take towards this person?

_____

_____

_____

_____

_____

_____

_____

_____

_____

_____

_____

_____

_____

_____

✦ When might you have pushed other people's boundaries? Even in simple scenarios like pushing them to join in on something when they'd already stated they couldn't do it.

_____

_____

_____

_____

_____

_____

_____

_____

_____

_____

_____

🌙 **ACTION:** Next time someone says 'no' to you, accept it instead of trying to convince them, this way you are showing that you respect their boundaries. And next time someone is trying to push your boundaries, make a mental note of it and consider whether this happens a lot with this person, and whether this person is actually good for you.

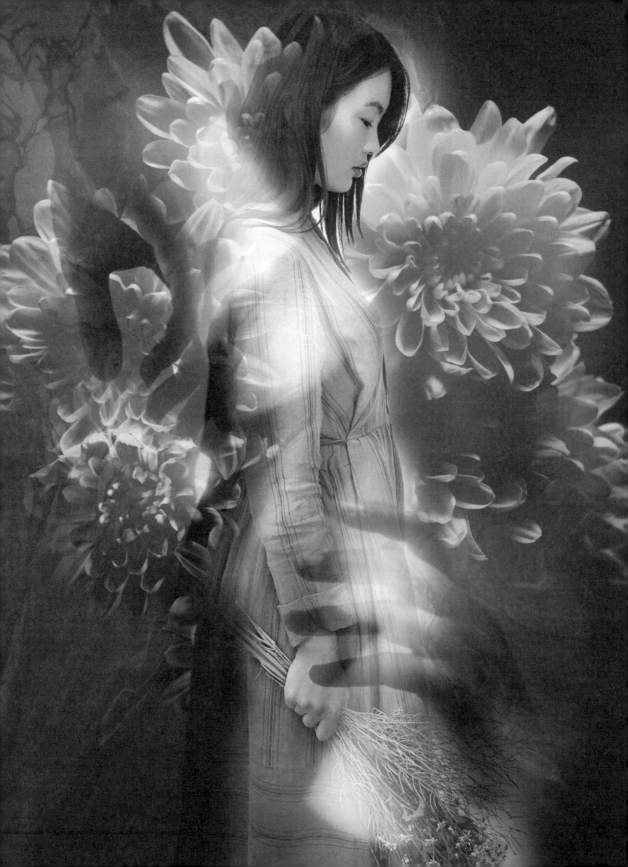

15. Apologising | Grudge

✦

AFFIRMATION:

'I am strong enough to admit my weakness.'

It might feel easier to hold a grudge towards someone you had a fight with rather than take responsibility for and own your part in contributing to the disagreement. You might have an inner battle of wanting to resolve the situation but hesitating to bring up the apology. There's often an internal push and pull; you want to resolve it but don't want to be the one taking the first step – it feels scary, humiliating, maybe even daunting.

✦ Initial thoughts:

_____

_____

_____

_____

_____

_____

_____

_____

What is the latest conflict you had with someone?

_____

_____

_____

_____

_____

_____

_____

What do you believe they did wrong?

_____

_____

_____

_____

_____

_____

_____

What is something unhelpful you said or did in the situation?

_____

_____

_____

_____

_____

_____

_____

_____

Change places with them in the situation. What might they have felt from what you did or said?

_____

_____

_____

_____

_____

_____

_____

◆ What can you do differently?

_____

_____

_____

_____

_____

_____

_____

◆ What steps can you take right now to resolve the conflict?

_____

_____

_____

_____

_____

_____

_____

_____

_____

ACTION: Write an apology letter to someone you have let down. You don't have to give them the letter or message yet, just use this as practice and perhaps with time it will feel easier to apologise when you do something wrong. The letter needs to include what you want to apologise for, what you did wrong and ask for forgiveness.

_____

_____

_____

_____

_____

_____

_____

_____

_____

_____

_____

_____

_____

_____

_____

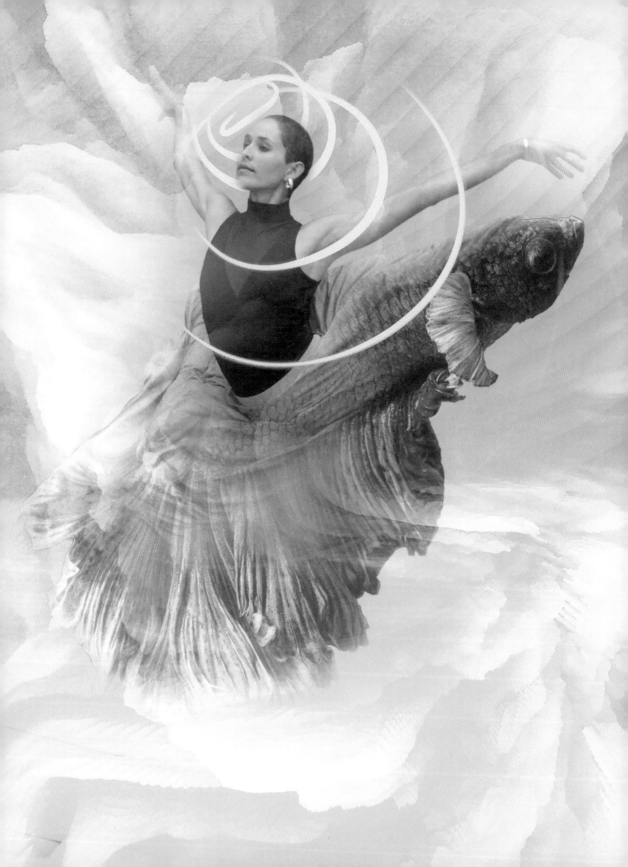

16. Behaviour | Interpretation

Behaviour is highly dependent on interpretation. We are intelligent beings and, therefore, how we behave is not simply a systemic reaction to what is happening around us. We have the ability to interpret, analyse and think before we take action. How we behave is a result of how we interpret the situation.

✦ Initial thoughts:

_____

_____

_____

_____

_____

_____

_____

✦ Think about a time when you got agitated about something someone said or
  did. Write about it here:

_____

_____

_____

_____

_____

_____

_____

_____

✦ What were the thoughts about them that came to your mind?

_____

_____

_____

_____

_____

_____

_____

✦ How can you challenge those thoughts?

_____

_____

_____

_____

_____

_____

_____

_____

✦ What could be some potential explanations as to why they behaved the way they did?

_____

_____

_____

_____

_____

_____

_____

_____

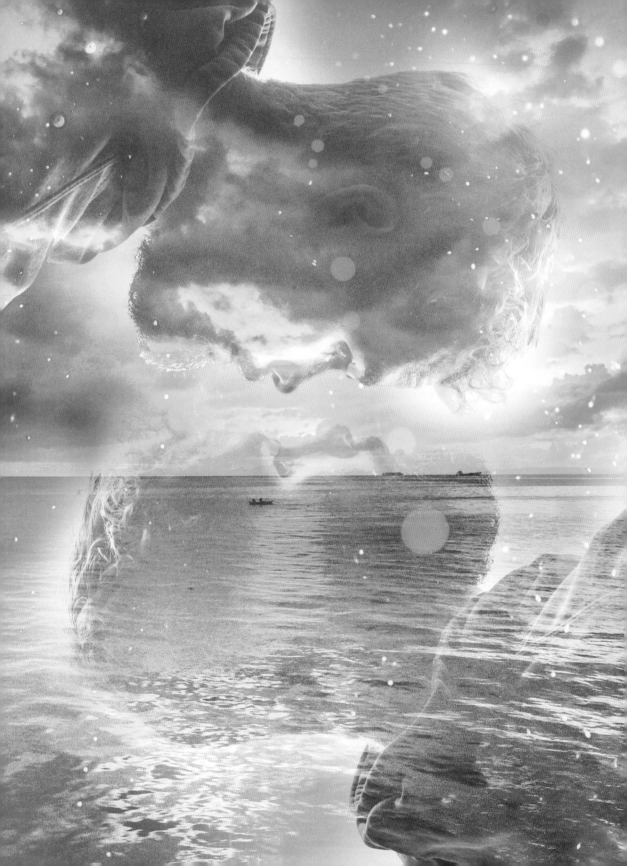

17. True self | Pseudo self

✦

AFFIRMATION:

'I am who I am and I don't need to make myself look better or worse than what I am.'

Life is a constant aim to find ourselves, be ourselves and show ourselves authentically to the world. But the reality is that we show many different versions of ourselves and not just one self. Sometimes we even show ourselves as someone we are not.

✦ Initial thoughts:

_____

_____

_____

_____

_____

_____

_____

_____

✦ What are the different selves you show to others? Who do you show to your friends? To your family? To your colleagues? To your partner? To strangers?

_____

_____

_____

_____

_____

_____

_____

_____

_____

_____

_____

_____

_____

_____

When do you feel like your most authentic self, and how does that reflect in your life currently?

_____

_____

_____

_____

_____

_____

_____

_____

_____

_____

_____

_____

_____

_____

✦ When challenged, how can you stay authentic and not make yourself seem either less or more than you are?

_____

_____

_____

_____

_____

_____

✦ When do you feel in need of other people's validation, approval or praise to feel good about yourself?

_____

_____

_____

_____

_____

_____

✦ How can you validate yourself instead?

_____

_____

_____

_____

_____

_____

_____

_____

_____

_____

_____

_____

🌙 **ACTION:** Next time you get the feeling that you want to show off, try and resist doing it if it isn't asked for.

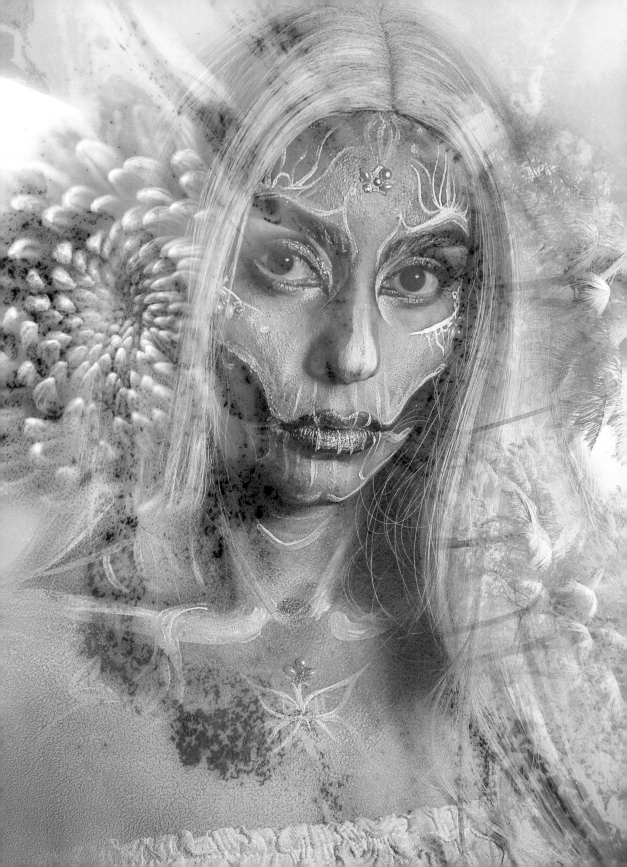

18. Forgiveness | Grimness

AFFIRMATION:

'I set myself free by forgiving . . .'

Forgiving someone doesn't make the thing they did to hurt you okay. Forgiving means setting yourself free of the pain someone has caused you. Forgiving someone is not for them, it's for you.

✦ Initial thoughts:

_____

_____

_____

_____

_____

_____

_____

_____

◆ What is something you have struggled to forgive someone for?

_____

_____

_____

_____

_____

_____

_____

_____

_____

_____

_____

_____

_____

_____

_____

✦ What pain might they have that has been passed to you?

_____

_____

_____

_____

_____

_____

_____

✦ What is a helpful thought you can tell yourself so you can let go of the pain?

_____

_____

_____

_____

_____

_____

_____

◆ How can forgiving them help you move forward?

_____

_____

_____

_____

_____

_____

_____

_____

◆ Do you feel the need to tell them you forgive them or can you tell yourself only?

_____

_____

_____

_____

_____

_____

_____

_____

ACTION: Whenever a grim thought about someone who hurt you comes up, practise repeating an affirmation and mantra that feels true for you in regard to the situation. For example:

'I forgive you, for you didn't know better.'

'I forgive you, but it doesn't make what you did acceptable.'

'I forgive you for me.'

'I forgive and let go; I don't let this inflict pain on me anymore.'

'I forgive you and wish you growth.'

Or write down your own:

_____

_____

_____

_____

_____

_____

_____

_____

_____

_____

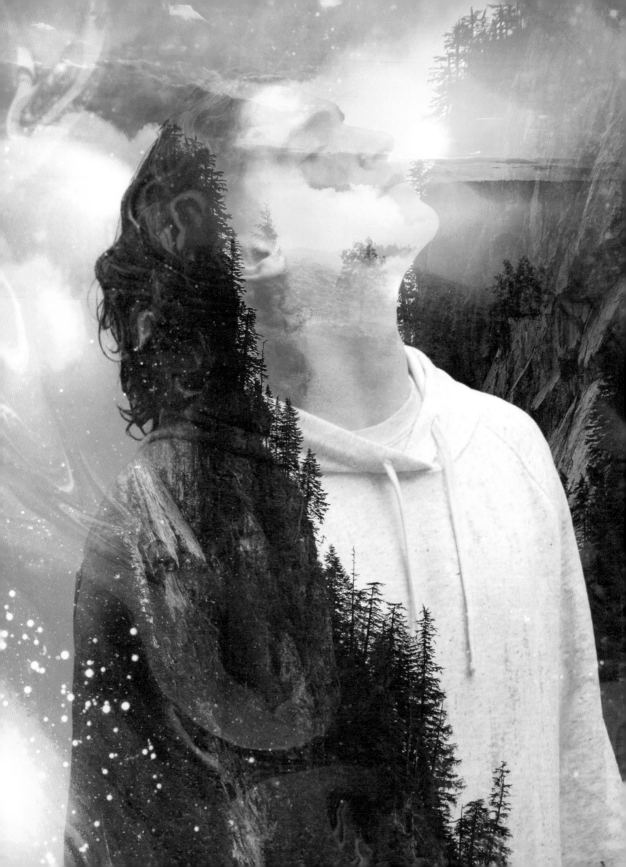

19. Solution | Problem

AFFIRMATION:

*'I have the power and ability
to change my situation.'*

There can be many different solutions to the same problem, but even so it's easy to feel stuck in whatever situation you are in, feeling that you don't have any options at all, that you don't have the ability to change your situation or to solve the problem you are facing right now.

✦ Initial thoughts:

_____

_____

_____

_____

_____

_____

_____

_____

What is a current problem you are facing?

_____

_____

_____

_____

_____

_____

_____

_____

What is your initial thought of a solution?

_____

_____

_____

_____

_____

_____

_____

_____

◆ What is an alternative solution?

_____

_____

_____

_____

_____

_____

_____

_____

◆ What have other people done in similar situations?

_____

_____

_____

_____

_____

_____

_____

_____

_____

◆ What is stopping you from taking action towards the solution?

_____

_____

_____

_____

_____

_____

_____

_____

◆ What do you need to make the solution happen?

_____

_____

_____

_____

_____

_____

_____

ACTION: Brainstorm ALL possible solutions with yourself no matter how crazy and scary and unrealistic they might feel. Write down every single solution you can think of on small, separate pieces of paper. Pick one at a time and put them into two piles – the 'No' pile and the 'Maybe' pile. Narrow down the 'Maybe' pile to the most feasible solution and you might find that you already had your answer within.

_____

_____

_____

_____

_____

_____

_____

_____

_____

_____

_____

_____

_____

_____

_____

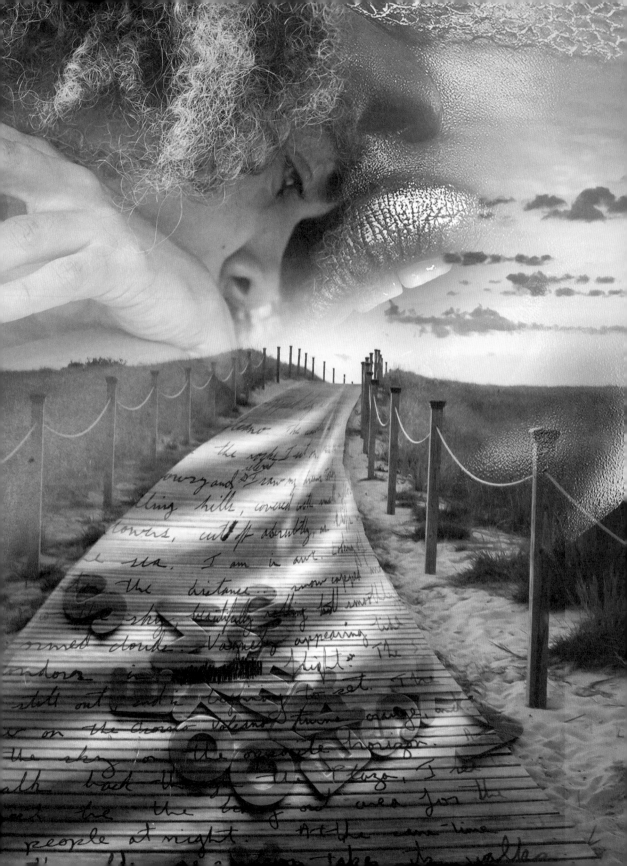

20. Energy | Motivation

✦

AFFIRMATION:

*'I should not do anything,
but I could do anything I want.'*

There are so many things in this world that easily drain both your energy and motivation to do things you might want to do. There are so many 'shoulds' being thrown around, both by others but also by you. How often have you heard yourself say, 'I should do this' and 'I should do that'? And not to mention the classic 'to-do list'. This feeling that we should but are not implies that what we currently are doing is not enough. This can lead to more stress and you might be even less likely to get things done.

✦ Initial thoughts:

_____

_____

_____

_____

_____

_____

_____

Make a list of all the 'shoulds' you currently feel, but swap the word 'should' to 'could'.

_____

_____

_____

_____

_____

_____

_____

_____

_____

_____

_____

_____

_____

◆ What other words cause you stress or pressure in your mind? What alternative, more neutral language could you use?

_____

_____

_____

_____

_____

_____

_____

_____

_____

_____

_____

🌙 **ACTION:** If you keep a to-do list, let's change it! Instead, make a must-not-do list or a could-do list.

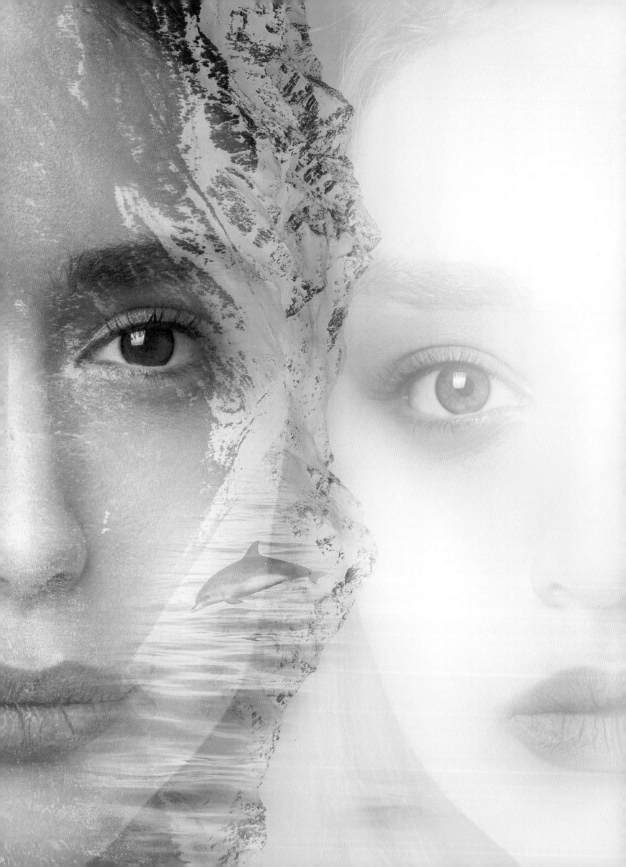

21. Asking | Telling

✦

AFFIRMATION:

'I show up to conversations to understand, not to prove I'm right.'

Asking questions and talking about our experiences are the fundamentals of conversations. They both have a place and they balance each other. If one or the other takes over, the conversation might lead down a narrow road especially when having a discussion, argument or misunderstanding with someone. See if you can show up to the conversation with a different view in mind: to understand rather than respond.

✦ Initial thoughts:

_____

_____

_____

_____

_____

_____

_____

_____

◆ When explaining your point of view to someone, how would you ideally like them to respond?

_____

_____

_____

_____

_____

_____

_____

_____

_____

_____

_____

_____

_____

_____

✦ Are you giving a similar response to others? What response do you usually give?

_____

_____

_____

_____

_____

_____

_____

_____

✦ Think about the last argument you had with someone. What could you have done differently to steer it into a conversation and understanding instead?

_____

_____

_____

_____

_____

_____

_____

_____

◆ What were your presumptions in that argument that you don't really have proof of?

_____

_____

_____

_____

_____

_____

_____

◆ What questions could you have asked to confirm if they were right or not?

_____

_____

_____

_____

_____

_____

_____

✦ For future interactions, note down what questions you can ask to gain more clarity before responding:

_____

_____

_____

_____

_____

_____

_____

✦ How can you open a conversation to encourage the other person to show understanding rather than coming up with solutions or arguing?

_____

_____

_____

_____

_____

_____

_____

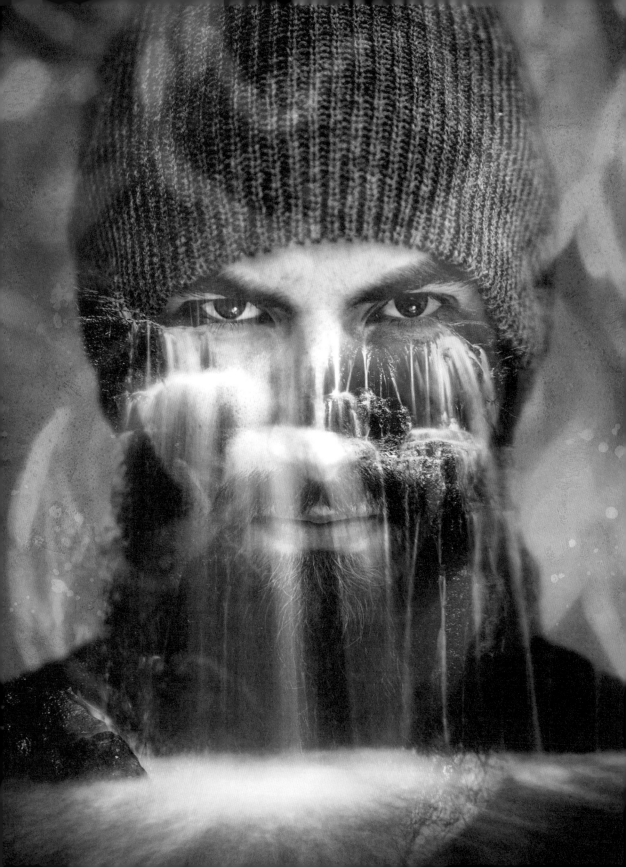

22. Sadness | Anger

AFFIRMATION:

'I use my anger as a guide to my inner depth.'

Sadness and crying are often seen or portrayed as weakness, whereas anger is often portrayed as a powerful and strong emotion. No wonder it's much easier to express anger instead of sadness. But the expression of anger is often just a shield to the underlying emotion of hurt. Anger is often used as a protective wall between you and other people. A shield to avoid showing your underlying vulnerability.

As anger and sadness are both powerful emotions, you can be sure that whenever these feelings arise there is something in the situation that deserves attention, and it is highly likely something that the person cares deeply about. Use this as a guide to find purpose and motivation both for yourself and others.

✦ Initial thoughts:

_____

_____

_____

_____

_____

_____

Think about the last time you were angry. What was the underlying feeling? Were you actually angry or were you feeling hurt?

_____

_____

_____

_____

_____

_____

_____

_____

How could you have expressed that more authentically instead of showing anger?

_____

_____

_____

_____

_____

_____

_____

◆ What are questions you can ask others when they express anger in order to understand the underlying cause?

_____

_____

_____

_____

_____

_____

_____

_____

_____

_____

_____

_____

_____

> 🌙 **ACTION:** Learn to ask questions about the hurt rather than the expression of anger. When someone is expressing anger or you find yourself expressing anger, throw out the question: 'What are you/am I feeling hurt about?'

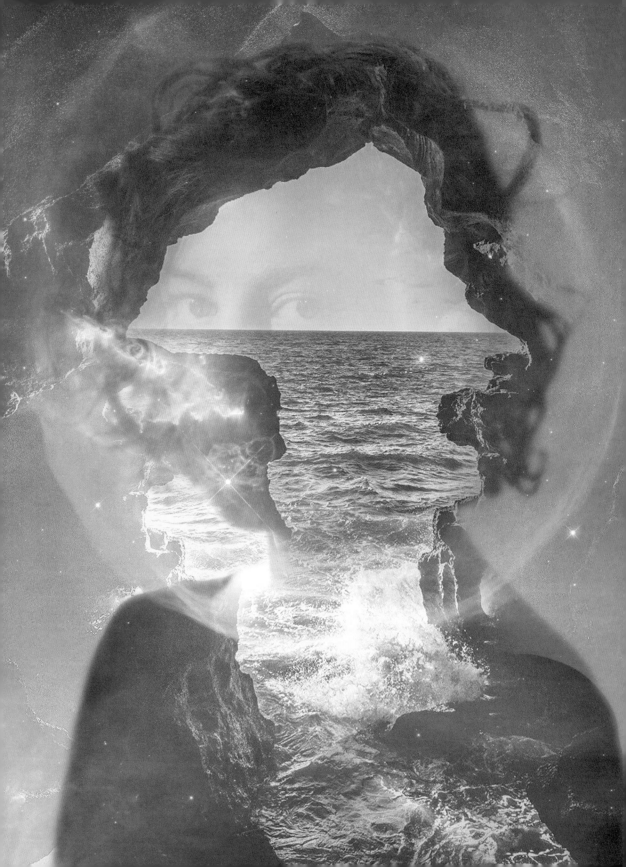

23. Obliviousness | Awareness

AFFIRMATION:

*'I am courageous enough to find out
whatever answers I need to hear.'*

Uncertainty plays a big factor in triggering anxiety. It can be uncertainty about your living situation, whether a person likes you or not, whether someone might leave you, whether you'll get the job you applied for, whether your boss will like your work . . . the list can go on and on! If you look at all these things and imagine a positive or a negative outcome, you might feel that the stress is not actually about the outcome itself but the fact that you don't know how things will turn out.

✦ Initial thoughts:

_____

_____

_____

_____

_____

_____

_____

What is something you are anxious about or find yourself ruminating on?

_____

_____

_____

_____

_____

_____

_____

What can you do to get a definite answer to these uncertainties?

_____

_____

_____

_____

_____

_____

_____

✦ Is there a decision you must make? If so, what do you need to be able to make that decision?

_____

_____

_____

_____

_____

_____

_____

_____

_____

_____

_____

_____

_____

🌙 **ACTION:** Collect your courage and take whatever action you need to get resolutions to your worries, and be prepared to hear whatever answer you might receive.

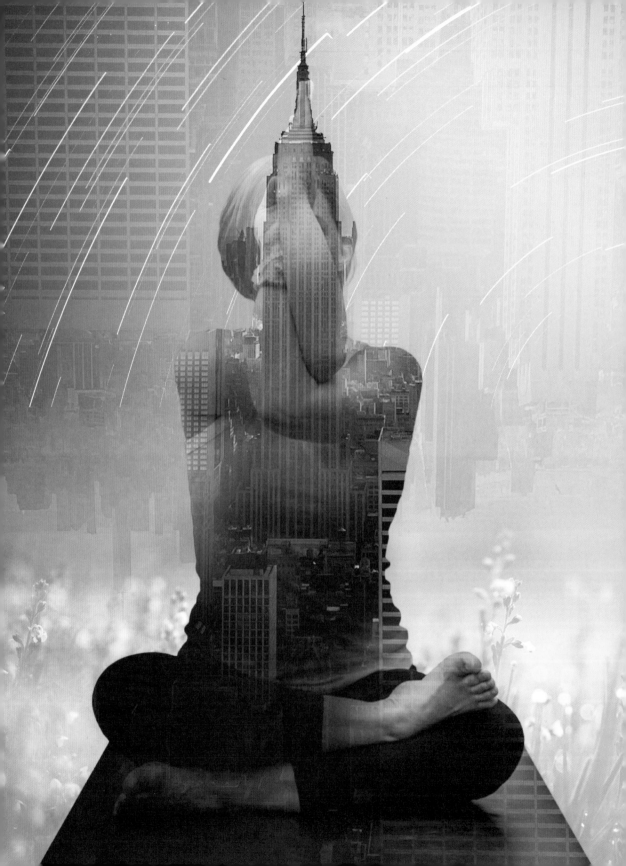

24. Meditation | Escapism

AFFIRMATION:

'I live and accept my own reality.'

It's common to believe that the purpose of meditation is to think about nothing, empty your mind and get a rest from your thoughts, your inner dialogue. But in reality, not to have any thoughts at all is nearly impossible as our brain is wired to do exactly that – think!

✦ Initial thoughts:

_____

_____

_____

_____

_____

_____

_____

_____

_____

◆ Note down what things you usually use to take a break from your thoughts. It might be watching TV, playing games, indulging in drugs or alcohol or anything else that takes up your focus:

_____

_____

_____

_____

_____

_____

_____

_____

_____

_____

_____

_____

_____

_____

♦ When do you usually find yourself resorting to these things?

_____

_____

_____

_____

_____

_____

_____

_____

_____

_____

_____

_____

_____

_____

_____

_____

◆ What thoughts are you trying to avoid?

_____

_____

_____

_____

_____

_____

_____

_____

_____

_____

_____

_____

_____

_____

_____

✦ What other ways can you address these thoughts instead of pushing them away?

_____

_____

_____

_____

_____

_____

_____

_____

_____

_____

_____

_____

☾ **ACTION:** Next time you feel the urge to run away from your thoughts, try and swap your go-to escape media for a guided meditation and see what happens. Guided meditations can be found in many different apps as well as online; do a quick search and see if you can find something that resonates with you.

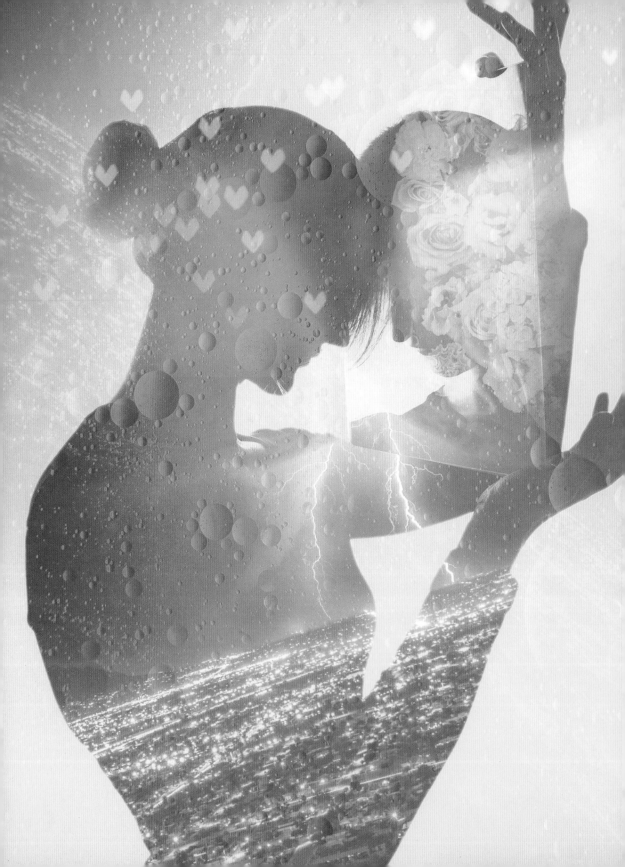

25. Self-love | Self-loathing

AFFIRMATION:

'I give myself permission to accept my imperfections.'

Self-loathing means putting yourself down and making yourself feel less than you are. It's the way you speak to yourself and the way you think about yourself. It is the opposite to self-love. Loving yourself doesn't mean you believe you are better than anybody else, but rather accepting you are not and believing that is okay.

✦ Initial thoughts:

_____

_____

_____

_____

_____

_____

✦ What are some examples in your life when you have sought love from others rather than from yourself?

_____

_____

_____

_____

_____

_____

_____

_____

✦ Are you currently having any negative thoughts about yourself? Look for thoughts that start with 'I am . . .' and finish in something negative or similar. List them here:

_____

_____

_____

_____

_____

_____

_____

◆ Take a moment to analyse these thoughts, are they true? What might be a different side or truth?

_____

_____

_____

_____

_____

_____

_____

◆ What are ways you can show yourself love?

_____

_____

_____

_____

_____

_____

_____

✦ List 3 things or more you love about yourself:

_____

_____

_____

_____

_____

_____

_____

✦ List 3 things or more that are not perfect about yourself but you now choose to accept:

_____

_____

_____

_____

_____

_____

_____

☾ ACTION: Make a poster to help remind you every day to show yourself love and appreciation. Take your favourite affirmation or any words you feel inspire you to love yourself more. Here are some suggestions:

'I am not perfect and I don't have to be.'

'I love and accept myself for who I am.'

'I am enough; I am worthy.'

Brainstorm your own ideas:

_____

_____

_____

_____

_____

_____

_____

_____

_____

_____

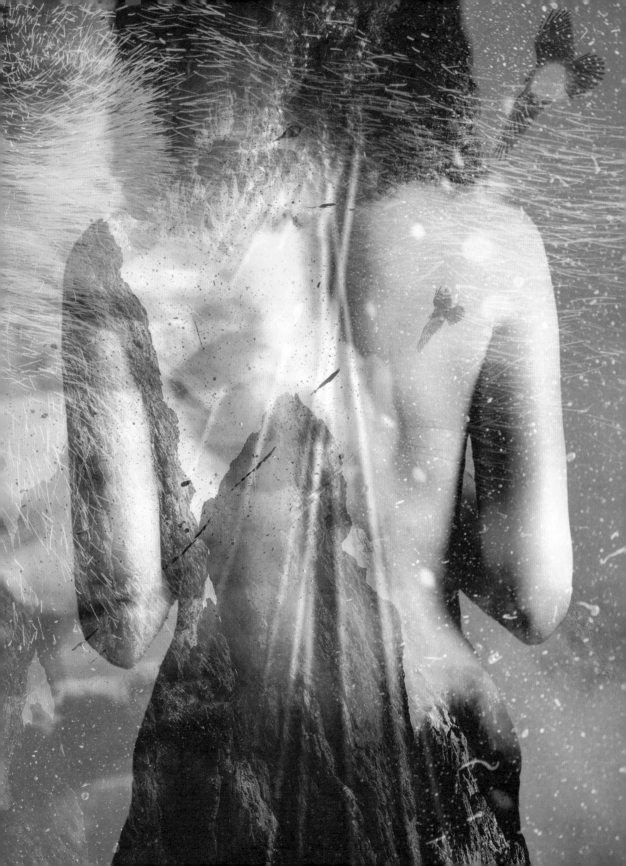

26. Fear | Anxiety

AFFIRMATION:

'I am afraid, but I will do it anyway.'

Anxiety is often caused by fear or worry about something that has not yet happened. It might never happen or it might not happen the way you think it will. And the part of not knowing and fearing the worst can cause an anxious and very uneasy feeling. On the contrary, after the event has happened, regardless of how it turned out, your anxiety will most likely ease if it was only tied to this specific event. So, the anxiety is not exactly related to the outcome, but the fact that the outcome is not known to us.

✦ Initial thoughts:

_____

_____

_____

_____

_____

_____

_____

_____

_____

Reflect on the things in your life that might feel uncertain now. What things do you currently not know the outcome of?

_____

_____

_____

_____

_____

_____

_____

_____

_____

_____

_____

_____

_____

_____

_____

What can you do to get clarity on the matter?

_____

_____

_____

_____

_____

_____

_____

_____

_____

_____

_____

_____

_____

_____

_____

_____

◆ What questions do you need to ask?

_____

_____

_____

_____

_____

_____

_____

_____

_____

_____

_____

_____

_____

_____

_____

_____

_____

List the actions you need to take to get an outcome:

_____

_____

_____

_____

_____

_____

_____

_____

_____

_____

_____

_____

_____

_____

_____

ACTION: To practise this, start with the smallest thing – whatever makes you the least anxious of the things you listed. Analyse what it is you need to do to gain clarity. Take action, put it in your calendar (ideally as soon as possible) and afterwards cross it off your list and take notice of how your feelings have changed.

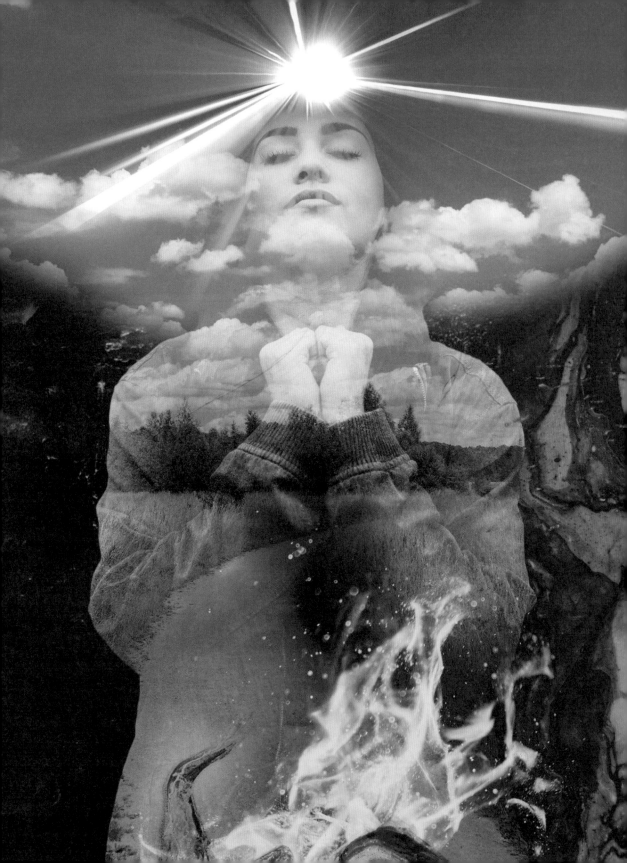

27. Offended | Enlightened

AFFIRMATION:

*'I don't waste my energy on the road of rage,
I stroll down the road of enlightenment.'*

Feeling offended by something is often a sign of an insecurity within yourself. It can cause a burning feeling in your stomach; you start to boil and arguments and things you'd like to defend yourself with pop into your mind. It can be truly exhausting so if you could learn to change your perspective you could save yourself a lot of energy. Noticing you are feeling offended can be used as a tool for yourself to find weak links that perhaps you need to work on.

✦ Initial thoughts:

_____

_____

_____

_____

_____

_____

◆ What are some things you have felt offended by recently?

_____

_____

_____

_____

_____

_____

_____

_____

_____

_____

_____

_____

_____

_____

_____

◆ Why did they make you feel offended?

_____

_____

_____

_____

_____

_____

_____

_____

_____

_____

_____

_____

_____

_____

◆ What feels true to you about the statements that made you feel offended?

_____

_____

_____

_____

_____

_____

_____

_____

◆ If you think about them more deeply, are they actually proven? What could be an alternative truth?

_____

_____

_____

_____

_____

_____

_____

ACTION: Next time you feel offended, make a note of it and once you've calmed down from the situation ask yourself the previous questions and make notes here.

_____

_____

_____

_____

_____

_____

_____

_____

_____

_____

_____

_____

_____

_____

_____

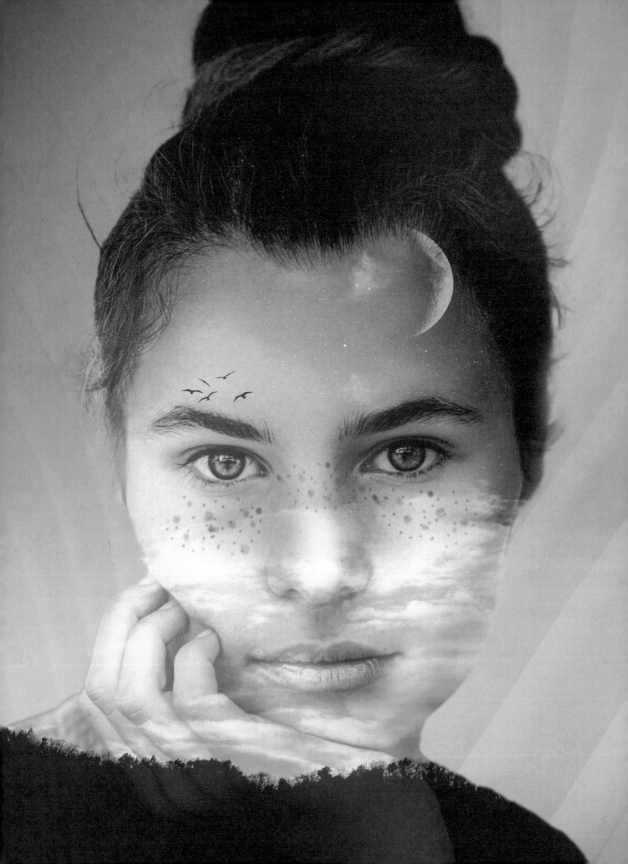

28. Freedom | Sacrifice

AFFIRMATION:

'I am free to make my dreams a reality.'

Most of us like to think of ourselves as free. We have the right and ability to choose how we live our lives. But even so a lot of people feel stuck in the situation they are in and only dream about where they wish to end up. However, freedom doesn't always come for free. True freedom, rather than just being able to do anything you want, is being able to choose what to sacrifice in order to live the life you want.

✦ Initial thoughts:

_____

_____

_____

_____

_____

_____

_____

_____

✦ What freedom would you like to have that you currently don't?

_____

_____

_____

_____

_____

_____

_____

✦ What do you need to sacrifice to achieve this freedom?

_____

_____

_____

_____

_____

_____

_____

◆ What steps do you need to take to be able to make these sacrifices?

_____

_____

_____

_____

_____

_____

WHAT DO YOU DREAM OF DOING BUT CURRENTLY FEEL YOU ARE UNABLE TO ACHIEVE?	
WHAT DO YOU HAVE TO SACRIFICE?	
STEPS YOU MUST TAKE TO BE ABLE TO MAKE THOSE SACRIFICES	

Start from the third row and work your way back through the steps; you'll be getting closer and closer to your true freedom.

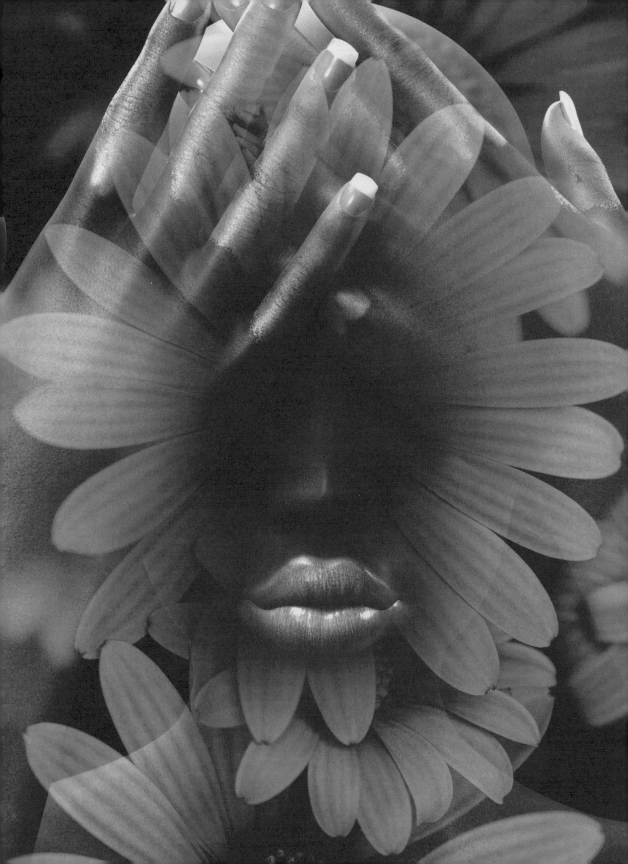

29. Cherishing | Suppressing

✦

AFFIRMATION:

'I cherish the beautiful moments that have been and take the lesson with me of the things that caused me pain.'

Instead of trying to forget things, what if you allowed yourself to cherish the good parts of what was and perhaps even accept the bad things? Suppressing emotions and memories doesn't necessarily make them go away. The pain might go away temporarily, but every time the memory is triggered you will relive it even more intensely.

✦ Initial thoughts:

_____

_____

_____

_____

_____

_____

What is something you would like to forget about?

_____

_____

_____

_____

_____

_____

_____

_____

What other things are you suppressing if you go a bit deeper?

_____

_____

_____

_____

_____

_____

_____

_____

_____

_____

How can you reframe these memories?

_____

_____

_____

_____

_____

_____

_____

_____

_____

What did you learn from them?

_____

_____

_____

_____

_____

_____

_____

_____

_____

_____

◇ What did you gain from them?

_____

_____

_____

_____

_____

_____

_____

◆ What would you have missed out on had they not happened?

_____

_____

_____

_____

_____

_____

_____

_____

ACTION: Find a belonging you have kept that brings out mixed emotions for you. Perhaps a gift from a loved one who is no longer in your life. Think about the memories it brings you, both the beautiful and the painful ones. See if you can neutralise the painful memories by giving them a different meaning.

For example, it might bring you pain because you are no longer with the person who gave you this gift, but because of how things turned out you might have learned something about yourself that can help you on your journey of love. Write down your thoughts here:

_____

_____

_____

_____

_____

_____

_____

_____

_____

_____

_____

_____

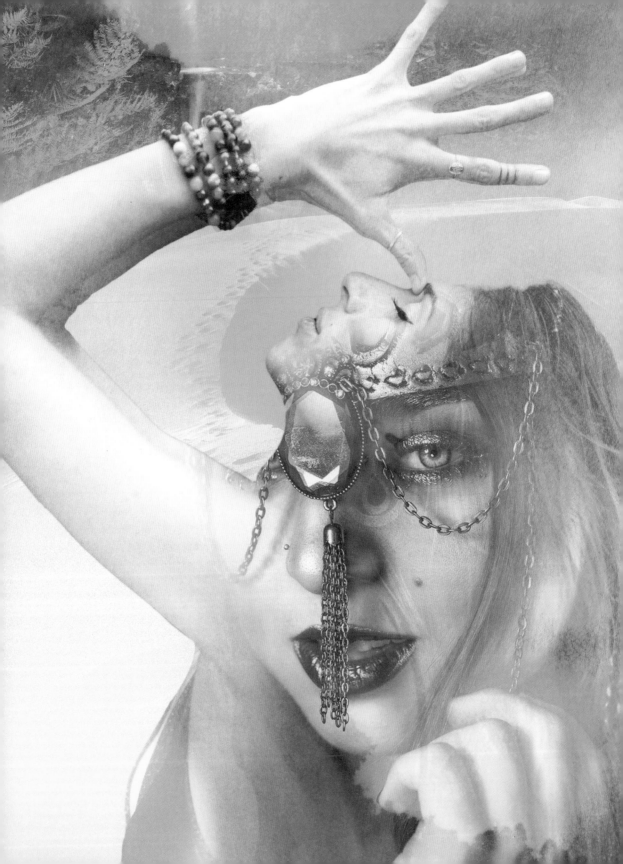

30. Appreciation | Greed

AFFIRMATION:

'I appreciate others and I appreciate myself.'

Have you ever felt that you don't get enough verbal appreciation and positive feedback yet receive a lot of negative comments? Maybe you can search within yourself and see if you can get the feelings of appreciation by giving to others what you are longing for.

✦ Initial thoughts:

_____

_____

_____

_____

_____

_____

_____

_____

_____

_____

What have you done recently to show appreciation for others?

_____

_____

_____

_____

_____

_____

What else can you do to show your love for the people in your life?

_____

_____

_____

_____

_____

_____

_____

What things would you like to be appreciated for? How can you give yourself appreciation for these?

_____

_____

_____

_____

_____

_____

_____

_____

_____

_____

_____

_____

_____

_____

List all the things you appreciate about yourself:

_____

_____

_____

_____

_____

_____

_____

_____

_____

_____

_____

_____

_____

_____

_____

◆ Make a list of your loved ones and note down what you appreciate about them. (Why not send them a message and let them know?)

_____

_____

_____

_____

_____

_____

_____

_____

_____

_____

_____

_____

_____

_____

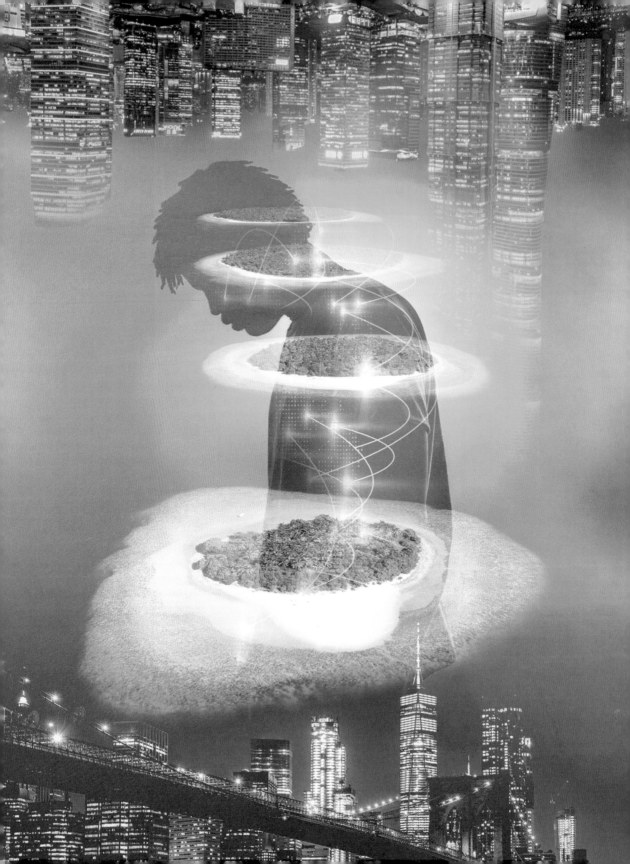

31. Loneliness | Connection

AFFIRMATION:

'I fill my heart and soul with meaningful connections.'

Feeling lonely isn't always caused by not having people around us, but by the lack of meaningful connections with the people in our lives. It can be helpful to look at the connections you have and see if there is anything you can do to improve them to make them deeper and more genuine. Connection with others is daring to give of yourself, showing that it is safe to share with you and that you welcome their true emotions and listen without judgement.

✦ Initial thoughts:

_____

_____

_____

_____

_____

_____

Who are the people you feel closest to at the moment, and why?

_____

_____

_____

_____

_____

_____

_____

_____

_____

_____

_____

_____

_____

_____

_____

What makes your relationship close?

_____

_____

_____

_____

_____

_____

_____

_____

_____

_____

_____

_____

_____

_____

_____

_____

Are there others who you wish you were closer with? Who are they, and why?

_____

_____

_____

_____

_____

_____

_____

_____

_____

_____

_____

_____

_____

_____

_____

What can you do to create a deeper connection with them?

_____

_____

_____

_____

_____

_____

_____

_____

_____

_____

_____

_____

ACTION: Choose the deeper questions in your conversations with the people you want to create a better connection with. Instead of focusing on surface questions and the facts of events, turn the focus onto their inner world. Ask about their thoughts and feelings and in the same manner, share yours with them.

179

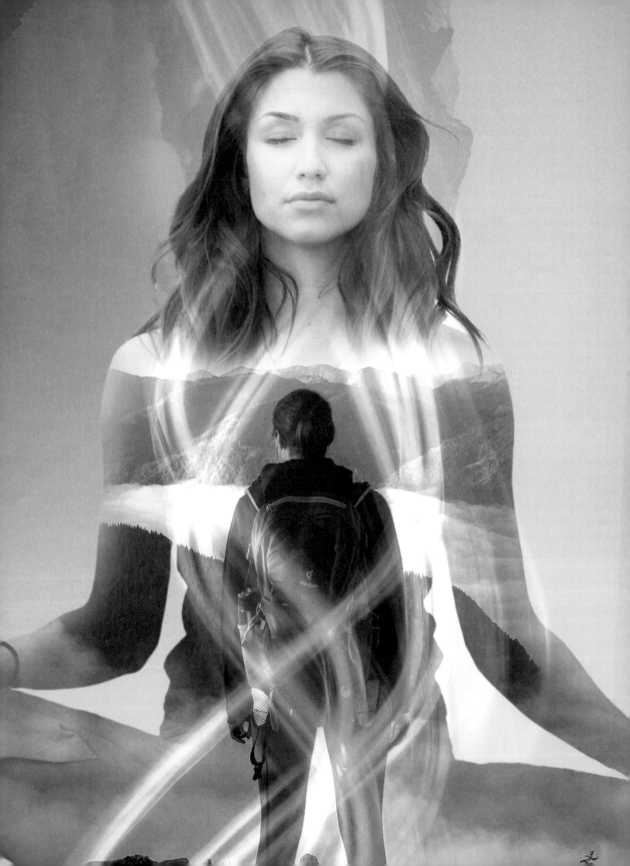

32. Relaxation | Activation

AFFIRMATION:

*'I let my emotional stress move
through and out of my body.'*

Not everything we think we know is true. And just because something cannot be proven, it doesn't mean it isn't there. If you are feeling uneasy, stressed or find it difficult to relax, know that it is not going to be there forever; things can change. Sometimes the best medicine for relaxation is activation. In order to be able to relax your mind, it can help that your body is also ready to do the same.

✦ Initial thoughts:

_____

_____

_____

_____

_____

_____

_____

_____

✦ What are some activities you enjoy that activate your body?

_____

_____

_____

_____

_____

_____

_____

_____

✦ List any activities that make you forget about time:

_____

_____

_____

_____

_____

_____

_____

_____

✦ What are some activities you haven't tried yet but might be interested in trying?

_____

_____

_____

_____

_____

_____

_____

_____

_____

🌙 **ACTION:** Choose an activity that you enjoy; it may be as simple as going for a walk or a more vigorous activity. While going through the motions, imagine your emotional pain or stress as fluid moving through your body with every movement.

If you are walking, visualise the feelings moving down to your legs and out through your feet. Or imagine your feelings as clouds evaporating from your body while moving through the exercises. Whatever feels right for you.

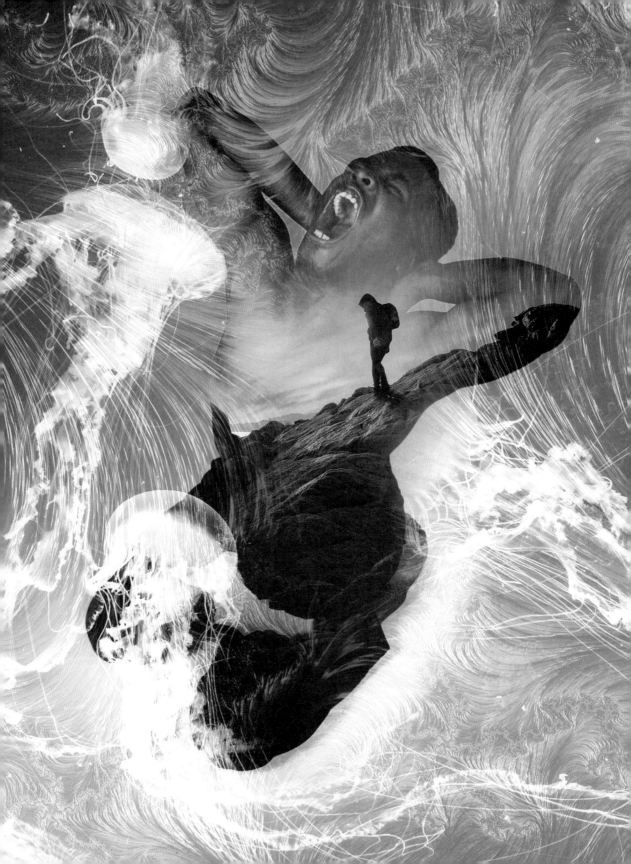

33. Action | Reaction

AFFIRMATION:

'I act rather than react.'

Action and reaction might seem like similar concepts, but there is one significant difference between the two. A reaction is an instant, almost impulsive response to something that is happening. An action, however, is a conscious decision made after consideration.

✦ Initial thoughts:

_____

_____

_____

_____

_____

_____

_____

_____

_____

Find your triggers. Take a week or two and every evening before going to bed, write down things that triggered you during the day. You can identify those triggers either by the physical feeling in your body or through ways you have reacted that you might have some regret about later. Note them down here:

_____

_____

_____

_____

_____

_____

✦ What pattern(s) can you see? For instance, is it always in relation to a certain topic, a certain person or perhaps a particular place?

_____

_____

_____

_____

_____

_____

_____

✦ What is your usual response in those situations?

_____

_____

_____

_____

_____

_____

_____

✦ What might be helpful for you to do when you feel triggered to delay your response? (Does it help you to go for a walk, visualise yourself in a different place, count to 10 or repeat a simple mantra or something else?) Choose a more helpful response to try next time it happens.

_____

_____

_____

_____

_____

_____

_____

_____

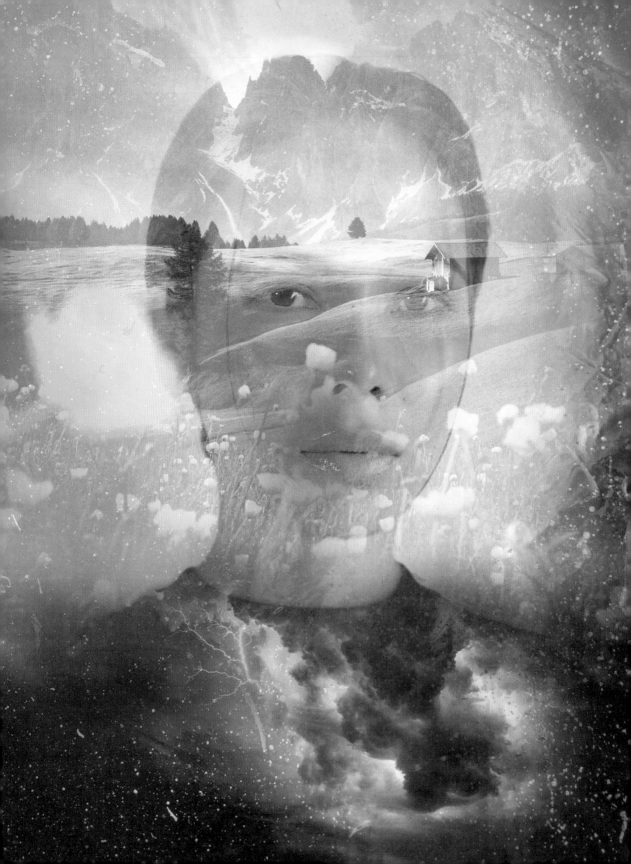

34. Conflict | Peace

'I face my conflict in order to restore peace.'

Sometimes a conflict needs to escalate in order to reach peace. You might be holding something in to avoid confrontation, but the longer it boils inside of you, the harder it becomes to hold it in. Eventually it will escalate to a conflict either by action or by confrontation. You might find that often after a conflict, the air has been cleared and peace is once again restored.

✦ Initial thoughts:

_____

_____

_____

_____

_____

_____

_____

_____

_____

_____

◆ If you have an issue that you need to resolve but are holding it in, write it down here:

_____

_____

_____

_____

_____

_____

_____

_____

◆ What mindset can you use to desensitise the issue in your own mind?

_____

_____

_____

_____

_____

_____

_____

◆ How can you bring up the issue in a non-threatening way with the goal to resolve and make it clear for everyone that there are good intentions and a call for peace and resolution, rather than conflict and fight?

_____

_____

_____

_____

_____

_____

_____

_____

_____

_____

_____

_____

_____

_____

_____

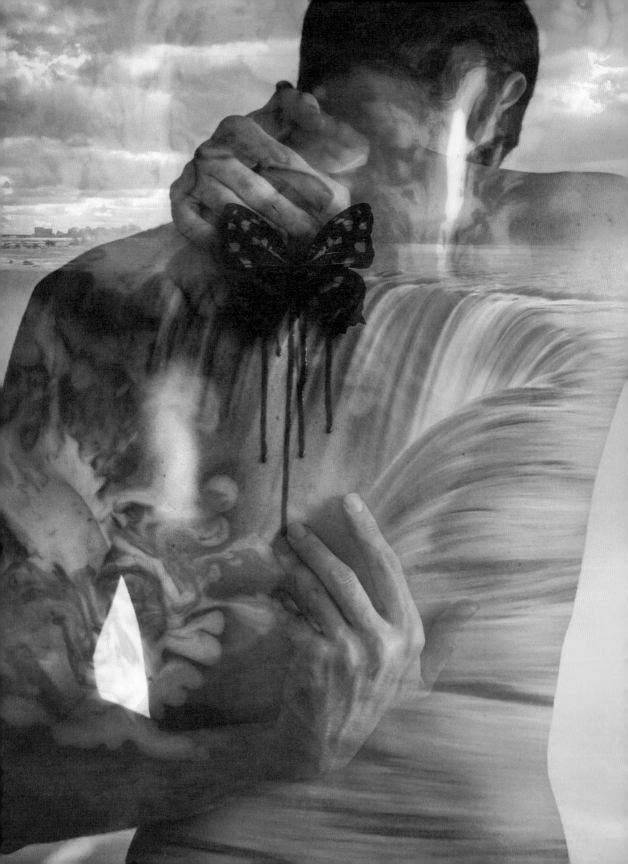

35. Physical pain | Emotional pain

Affirmation:

'I am calm; I am grounded; I am safe.'

Your body and mind are highly connected and your nervous system runs through your whole body. If you have ever experienced a gut feeling, it is a very strong confirmation that your body knows what is going on emotionally or cognitively. Emotional pain can manifest in your body and show up as physical pain. Especially if there is something troubling you that you have been ignoring for a long time. If you are experiencing difficult situations, try to be mindful of what it feels like in your body, whether it's pressure over your heart, a tight stomach or something else. Stress is a common factor in causing physical pain, so it is always good to be mindful and manage stress in your life.

✦ Initial thoughts:

_____

_____

_____

_____

_____

_____

◆ What physical pain are you currently experiencing?

_____

_____

_____

_____

_____

_____

_____

◆ What is the relation of this to any emotional pain?

_____

_____

_____

_____

_____

_____

_____

_____

◆ When does the the physical pain show up — in certain situations or is it constantly there?

_____

_____

_____

_____

_____

_____

◆ When is the pain most prominent?

_____

_____

_____

_____

_____

_____

_____

_____

◆ Have you noticed any things that ease the pain for you or make you forget about it?

_____

_____

_____

_____

_____

_____

_____

_____

_____

_____

_____

_____

_____

_____

✦ What can you do to minimise stress in your life?

_____

_____

_____

_____

_____

_____

_____

_____

_____

_____

_____

_____

_____

☾ **ACTION:** Minimise stress by giving yourself some love, care and acceptance. Use the calming sensation of a hot bath and visualise and repeat in your mind: 'This water calms my body and mind.' Play some music that you like and imagine the sound waves vibrating your pain away or take a shower and imagine the water washing away the pain from your body.

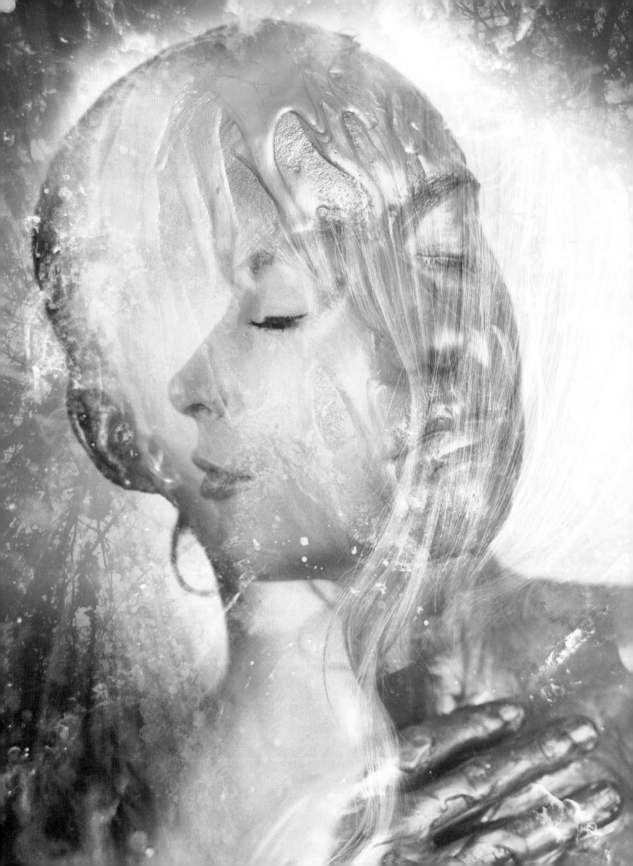

36. Gratitude
| Indulgence

✦

AFFIRMATION:

'I feel grateful; I am grateful.'

Gratitude is one of the best concepts to practise in order to live a happy and fulfilled life. It's easy to become lost in indulgence and try to acquire more and more – be it more things, more friends, more money or more fame. Here's a chance for you to acknowledge and appreciate what you have.

✦ Initial thoughts:

_____

_____

_____

_____

_____

_____

_____

_____

_____

What are the major things in your life that you appreciate the most?

_____

_____

_____

_____

_____

_____

_____

_____

_____

_____

_____

_____

_____

_____

✦ Make a list of things you are grateful for in your life (you can add to this list every day or as often as you want; try and acknowledge the little things in your day-to-day life):

_____

_____

_____

_____

_____

_____

_____

_____

_____

_____

_____

_____

_____

☾ **ACTION:** Start a daily gratitude journal. Get a new journal dedicated to this topic only. Write down at least one thing every day, or as often as you can, that you feel grateful for. Write as many as you can think of or if you are struggling write down one thing. Feel free to repeat what you were grateful for yesterday if it still feels true for you.

SUMMARISING – ACKNOWLEDGE YOUR GROWTH

Use these pages to reflect on the areas that you have worked on and acknowledge the growth you've experienced. Reflect on things such as where you feel you have grown the most. What has been the most helpful? What are you most grateful for on this journey? What are the biggest improvements you have made?

_____

_____

_____

_____

_____

_____

_____

_____

_____

_____

_____

_____

_____

_____

_____

_____